COMPLETE TRIATHLON BOOK

Triathlete magazine's

COMPLETE TRIATHLON BOOK

THE TRAINING, DIET, HEALTH, EQUIPMENT, AND SAFETY TIPS YOU NEED TO DO YOUR BEST

MATT FITZGERALD

WELLNESS CENTRAL

NEW YORK   BOSTON

Wellness Central
Hachette Book Group
237 Park Avenue
New York, NY 10017
Visit our Web site at www.HachetteBookGroup.com.

Wellness Central is an imprint of Grand Central Publishing
The Wellness Central name and logo are trademarks of Hachette Book Group, Inc.

Printed in the United States of America

First Edition: March 2003
10 9 8 7

Library of Congress Catalog-in-Publication Data

Fitzgerald, Matt.
    Triathlete magazine's complete triathlon book : the training, diet, health, equipment,
and safety tips you need to do your best / Matt Fitzgerald.
        p. cm.
    Includes index.
    ISBN 978-0-446-67928-2
    1. Triathlon. I. Triathlete. II. Title.

GV1060.73 .F58 2003
796.42'57--dc21   2002027233

Book design: HRoberts Design

In memory of Ryan Niles, who embodied the spirit of triathlon.

Contents

Foreword

During my 15-year career in triathlon I tried just about every exotic training technique and philosophy available. But I always came back to the few simple methods and principles that, when executed over and over and over, made the crucial difference between a good finish and a great one. Simpler was always better.

I liked the idea of following a program that was so complicated, I felt I needed a graduate degree just to decipher it. The searching side of me thought if I could barely understand the training schedule it must be good for me. But the practical side of me, which cared only for effectiveness, knew that a small handful of proven training practices applied day after day was the factor that would separate me from my competitors at the finish line.

This is not to say that I did not keep learning and refining my approach throughout my career, because I did. This is where my searching side came in handy. It drove me to continually try new means in the quest for improvement, while my practical side made sure that I carefully scrutinized each of them and kept only what worked.

The result of this approach, combining simplicity and exploration, when applied with a good amount of consistency, was six wins at the Hawaii Ironman World Championship and titles at virtually every other major event on the planet. I'm pleased to say that this same philosophy is reflected in a clear, comprehensive and useful way in *Triathlete Magazine's Complete Triathlon Book*. I firmly believe it is the best philosophy not just for world champions but for everyone who seeks improvement and enjoyment in the sport of triathlon.

This book does more than simply tell you how to prepare your body.

Its broad-based approach will give you the tools you need to do everything, from selecting and using equipment to preparing mentally for competition. I am confident you will see that the information in the pages ahead will not only help you go from the first step in training to success in racing, but will also take you on a journey of personal growth through the world of sports.

So dive in. Find out what really works in training. Explore what it means to be alive through competition and how great the journey to the start line really can be. Set in motion the plan that will take you to the exhilaration of seeing the finish line banner coming into sight!

Triathlete has long been a leader and authority in the sport. And above all, it has helped countless men and women of all ages around the world celebrate life through their own personal victory in triathlon. This book is long overdue and is everything I could have hoped for from such a trusted source. Enjoy it start to finish.

Mark Allen

Introduction

A few years back, *Triathlete* ran a monthly department called "My First Triathlon" in several consecutive issues. We invited our readers to write down and submit the story of their first triathlon experience—whether pleasant or painful, triumphal or tragic, or even comedic. Each month, we selected a particularly interesting story and published it. When we came up with the idea for this department, we expected to receive just enough submissions to constitute a legitimate contest.

We got a flood of submissions. And in retrospect, we should have anticipated it, because we, the staff of the magazine, had all done first triathlons ourselves, and they had changed our lives, just as the lives of the hundreds of our readers who wrote to us had been changed by their own experiences. This was the one theme that recurred in every single story we received. The details were always different. Some readers suffered hugely in their first triathlon, while others coasted. Some went fast, others went slow. Some got hooked sometime during the race itself, while others realized they were hooked only after they'd crossed the finish line. But they all got hooked.

You can't ever forget your first triathlon. Nor can you go through the process of preparing for a triathlon without experiencing a transformation both physical and mental. And it's all good. You become fitter than you've ever been, you look great, you feel great, and you start to enjoy using your body like you haven't done since you were a kid. At the same time, you develop discipline and focus, you gain confidence, and when you do cross that first finish line, you receive an infusion of good old-fashioned self-respect that can never be taken away from you. Nor does it end there. Being a triathlete is a journey of discovery that rewards you as long as you care to pursue it. People ask me all the time why I do triathlons, and train so hard for them. These are the things I tell them.

If you've done one or more triathlons, you know what I'm talking about. If you're preparing for your own first triathlon, you'll understand what I'm talking about in due time. In either case, this book is for you. Its aim is to provide you with all the information, perspective, and motivation you need to reap the many benefits of the triathlon lifestyle in the fullest measure for as long as you care to receive them.

It all begins with a simple goal: to swim, bike, and run your way from a starting line to a finish line as fast as you are able. It is in the process of pursuing this simple goal that all the real rewards of being a triathlete are gathered. On one level, this book is all about helping you become faster. In it, I will show you how to select and use equipment for speed, how to construct a training program that will maximize your fitness (hence your speed) for your next big race, how to fuel your body for performance, and so forth.

On another level, though, the pages that follow are equally concerned with helping you derive the greatest possible enjoyment from the whole triathlon experience. And so, at the end of each of the book's ten chapters, you'll find a special section that's strictly lifestyle-related, and in Chapter 9, "Mental Training," I'll spend as much time talking about such things as balancing your pursuit of triathlon with your important relationships as I do about matters like overcoming pre-race nerves. I just don't think any triathlon book could call itself "complete" without addressing the sport in its proper context—your life!

Yet this is not a fluffy book. I have written with the highly competitive triathlete in mind as much as the beginner. It wasn't difficult, either, because the same general principles and methods apply to all triathletes, from the back of the pack to the front. Every triathlete wants to improve. Lasting improvement comes when you are able to consistently learn from your training and racing experiences and use this knowledge to refine your future preparation and execution. More than mere information, this ability depends on a certain kind of *experimental* approach to the sport that, in my experience, even most veteran triathletes lack. Only when you have the tools you need to keep learning from and refining your pursuit of triathlon are you truly in control of your development as a triathlete. If this book has a training philosophy, I just stated it. I want to put you in control—real control—as a triathlete, whether you're an anxious newbie or a trash-talking stud (see "Triathlon Slang" on page 128) looking for a final edge.

If you have any questions, e-mail me: fitwriter@hotmail.com. Otherwise, I hope to see you on the starting line!

CHAPTER 1

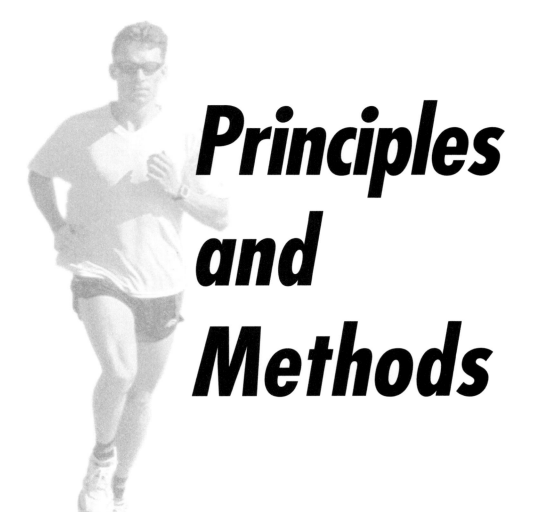

Principles and Methods

*I*n 1978, a small but spirited group of endurance athletes completed
the first Ironman Triathlon (2.4-mile swim, 112-mile bike, 26.2-mile run),
just to see whether they could. The following year, many of the same athletes and a few new joiners completed a second Ironman, just to see
whether they could do it *better*. What made these early triathletes confident that they *could* do better was the fact that they were able to try different ways of preparing for the second Ironman based on what had
been learned in preparing for and attempting the first. For some of the
participants, this was as simple a matter as swimming, cycling, *and* running in the months preceding the race, rather than doing just one of the
three! This pattern of practical and incremental learning continued to
unfold as the number and variety of triathlon events and participants
rapidly multiplied over the ensuing years. Such has been the evolution
of the art of triathlon training.

"In the beginning, we really had no idea what we were doing," says
triathlon legend Mark Allen, who did his first Ironman in 1982. "There
was very little information available about how to train for three sports
at such distances." Allen and the other first-generation triathletes gradually chipped away at this information gap by borrowing various training
practices from swimmers, cyclists, runners, and one another, and retain-
ing only those that worked best.

Today, thanks to the efforts of Allen and his peers, triathlon training
is fairly standardized. We now have a comprehensive set of established
principles and proven methods of training that take much of the guess-

work out of the process. Many triathletes still defy these guidelines, through ignorance in some cases and head-strongness in other cases, but the consequences are always bad. Yet this is not to say that all wise triathletes train the same. The framework of guidelines is not so narrowly defined that there isn't room for distinct training philosophies, and furthermore, one of the established rules of triathlon preparation is that training must be customized to the individual. This is one of the reasons that understanding the principles and methods of triathlon training is so important—it gives you a foundation to support your own training decisions. It allows you to take true ownership of your development as a triathlete.

I have distilled the established principles and proven methods of triathlon training into eight rules, which I will now share with you in a sensible order. The present chapter will remain fairly general and abstract. In subsequent chapters, I will show you more specifically how to apply these rules concretely to *your* training and racing.

Rule #1: Train for Endurance

Endurance is the ability to perform relatively intense work over an extended period of time, or, put another way, the ability to delay the onset of fatigue. Because even the shortest triathlons take at least an hour for the fastest athletes to complete, triathlon is duly classified as an endurance sport. Therefore, triathlon training is mostly about maximizing endurance.

What gives a well-trained triathlete the ability to swim, bike, and run at a fairly high rate of speed for a long time? There are two key factors. Above all it is the ability to conserve an energy source called *glycogen* that allows the well-trained triathlete to swim, bike, and run far. And above all, it is the ability to rapidly transport oxygen to the working muscles to metabolize glycogen and other fuels that allows the well-trained triathlete to maintain a high rate of speed while going far. Here's why.

The human body is capable of two forms of energy metabolism, *aerobic* and *anaerobic*. The specific form that predominates at any given time is determined by the *intensity* of the movements being performed by the body. Intensity is basically the rate at which your body is burning energy during exercise (which is closely correlated with rate of speed in swimming, cycling, and running).

In aerobic metabolism, oxygen drawn from the atmosphere is used to burn mostly carbohydrate and fat for energy. The advantage of aerobic metabolism is that it can continue for quite a long time—how long depends on the precise intensity. Its disadvantage is that 60 to 80 seconds are required to create usable energy in this way, and so aerobic metabolism cannot support work of the highest intensities (such as sprinting).

To supply energy for very high-intensity movements, the body relies on anaerobic metabolism, in which carbohydrate is broken down without the use of oxygen. The advantage of this system is that it provides energy far more quickly and efficiently than aerobic metabolism. Its disadvantage is that glycogen breakdown without oxygen results in rapid production of the compound *lactic acid* (also called lactate), which accumulates in the blood and inhibits movement.* As anyone who has experienced it can attest, working above this *anaerobic threshold,* or *lactate threshold,* produces the sensation that one's muscles are spontaneously turning into pudding.

It's not an all-or-nothing threshold. When you're exercising between the anaerobic threshold and all-out sprint intensity, your body gets some of its energy aerobically and some of it anaerobically. It uses all the oxygen available and lets the lactate system take up the slack. But you can go a lot further when working just below the anaerobic threshold, where your body can clear away lactic acid as fast as your muscles produce it, than you can go when working just above the threshold, where the balance turns in favor of lactate. There's not a triathlete on earth who can sustain an anaerobic effort long enough to complete even a short triathlon. Hence, the faster you can swim, bike, and run while remaining *below* this all-important threshold, the faster you can do a triathlon. It all depends on how rapidly your body can supply oxygen to the muscles for fuel metabolism.

The best way to enhance your body's capacity for oxygen delivery and lactate clearance, and to thereby increase your anaerobic threshold, is by spending a lot of time training beneath the anaerobic threshold and somewhat less time training right at or just slightly above it. This kind of training increases lactate transporters in the blood and stimulates a variety of physiological adaptations that assist in oxygen delivery: a stronger heart, thicker blood, more "aerobic" enzymes in the muscle cells, and so forth. This explains the importance of oxygen delivery to endurance. Now, how about conserving glycogen?

It's like this. Your body can break down carbohydrate, protein, and fat for fuel. Protein is the body's least preferred energy source because

---

* The body produces lactic acid at lower intensity exercise, too (and even at rest), but at these lower intensities it can be cleared from the blood as fast as it is produced.

5

muscle tissue must be destroyed in order to release protein energy. This only happens in any significant amount late in workouts when the body is getting desperate. The human body has an almost boundless supply of fat fuel.[*] However, releasing energy from fat is slightly less efficient than releasing fat from carbohydrate, so the body tends to burn carbohydrate preferentially for energy during exercise, especially at higher intensities. Also, the body cannot burn fat alone, but must always burn it with a small amount of carbohydrate, whose supply is much more limited than the fat supply. A well-trained endurance athlete working just below the anaerobic threshold will see his or her carbohydrate fuel stores more or less depleted in about two and a half hours, at which point the athlete will be completely exhausted and unable to continue. Carbohydrate depletion is therefore almost always the cause of exhaustion in aerobic-intensity exercise.

Endurance training enhances the body's ability to store and conserve carbohydrate fuel. If you consistently do longer workouts that deplete these stores, your body will respond by stashing away more carbohydrate between workouts. Your body will also adapt to these longer workouts by producing more fat-burning enzymes, enhancing your body's ability to use fat for fuel. This will decrease the rate at which you burn carbohydrate during aerobic exercise and greatly increase the duration you're able to continue it.

Carbohydrate depletion is considered to be the primary agent of fatigue in endurance sports, but there are two others. One of them is central nervous system fatigue (commonly referred to as *central fatigue*). Unlike your muscles, your brain gets its energy exclusively from glucose. When your blood glucose level drops during extensive exercise, a biochemical chain reaction occurs that results in a shift in the balance of certain hormones in your brain. The result is simply that you start to feel miserable and lose the urge to continue, and at the same time, the neural signals telling your limbs to move are inhibited. These symptoms generally emerge at the same time as muscle fatigue, because they share a root cause (depletion of carbohydrate fuel). Hence, the same training methods that extend muscle endurance also extend the endurance of the central nervous system. But you can also limit the psychological component of central fatigue by developing the mental skills needed to overcome late-race suffering.

A final endurance limiter is muscle tissue breakdown. During exercise, the working muscles suffer microscopic tearing. The longer you go,

---

* Incidentally, at rest your muscles burn fat for energy almost exclusively.

How Endurance Training Affects the Body

Following are the major, performance-related physiological changes that occur as a result of endurance training. This list does not include all known adaptations, nor is the list of known adaptations itself considered to be complete.

Nervous System
Neural pathways develop between the brain and the most repetitively used motor units in the muscles, allowing for more efficient and coordinated movements of the kinds most often practiced.

Muscles
The muscles store greater amounts of glycogen (carbohydrate fuel), triglyceride (fat fuel), and myoglobin (a protein that stores oxygen). These adaptations increase the body's ability to produce energy. The number of mitochondria in the muscle cells increases. As the mitochondria are the site of aerobic metabolism, this adaptation increases oxygen consumption capacity. The size and possibly the number of muscle fibers increase in some muscles. These changes result in greater muscle strength.

Heart
The heart muscle becomes larger and more powerful, hence capable of pumping more blood per contraction. Consequently, the resting pulse rate decreases, as well as the heart rate associated with any given level of intensity in exercise.

Blood
Blood plasma volume and hemoglobin content increase, improving your body's ability to carry oxygen to the muscles.

Vascular System
Capillary density in the muscles increases. Capillaries deliver oxygen from the bloodstream to the muscles, so this adaptation also increases the body's capacity to consume oxygen.

Body Fat
The muscles metabolize more fat both at rest and at moderate levels of exercise. This adaptation increases endurance and decreases levels of stored body fat, which puts the athlete at an ideal race weight.

Bones
The density of many bones increases, making them stronger and more injury-resistant.

Linhchi Tang

the more such damage accumulates, the more sore your muscles feel, and the less healthy tissue you have left with which to keep moving. Further damage to the muscles occurs when carbohydrate fuel runs low and the body begins breaking down more muscle protein for energy. Consistent aerobic training with periodic long workouts makes the muscle tissue more resilient against tearing and also delays the use of protein for energy.

Beyond all this biochemistry, another big factor in the endurance equation is what's called *efficiency*. In triathlon, efficiency refers to the amount of energy that is required to maintain a given pace in swimming, biking, or running. Clearly, less is better, because the less fuel you burn now, the more you'll have left later. Efficiency happens on two levels. One is neuromuscular. By repeating certain movements over and over in training, and at the same time varying these movements in certain ways (running both uphill and downhill, fast and slow, for example), your brain learns to eliminate waste from the movement signals it sends to your muscles and also to distribute the workload among a greater number of motor units within your muscles. The other level of efficiency is technique. Good technique in swimming, cycling, and running is that which maximizes power production while minimizing the associated energy cost. For example, rotating the body from side to side during swimming reduces water drag and allows one to swim with less energy output. Triathletes can improve their technique by doing an appropriate amount of training at a fast pace, because form tends to improve as speed increases, and by performing special technique drills in each discipline.

The last thing I'd like to say about the nature of endurance is that it is highly task-specific. For example, training exclusively in swimming will make you only marginally better as a cyclist. This is because, by swimming, your body will learn to transport oxygen more rapidly mostly to the muscles used in swimming, will increase glycogen storage in these same muscles, and will increase efficiency only in the swimming movement patterns. Therefore, as a triathlete you need to maintain a consistent balance of training in swimming, cycling, and running in order to improve in all three.

Rule #2: Train Specifically

One of the more commonsensical rules of triathlon training is that it must be as specific as possible to the demands of racing. Put another way, triathlon training needs to closely model the various circumstances of racing, because only by doing this can you stimulate the physical adaptations needed to prepare your body for an optimal race effort.

Of course, there is a limit to how closely one can simulate racing in training. Performing a maximum-effort simulated triathlon every day is not the best way to prepare for an actual triathlon. There is more than one reason this doesn't work, but the main reason is that you can become better prepared for a triathlon by separating the various demands that racing places on the body and preparing for each of them individually. By compartmentalizing in this way, you can stimulate more pronounced adaptations of the kinds needed for an optimal race performance. For example, by doing a certain amount of your training in each discipline at a faster pace than you could ever maintain in an actual race, you can stimulate greater improvement in your efficiency in each discipline. At the same time, by doing a certain number of swim, bike, and run workouts that are longer than the swim, bike, and run segments of your next triathlon, you can develop greater endurance in each discipline.

The most basic application of the principle of specificity has to do with training volume. The longer the triathlon you're training for, the more training you need to do in order to develop the endurance you'll need to finish it or to achieve the time goal you've set for it. The principle of specificity also applies to the balance of training you perform among the three triathlon disciplines. In a typical triathlon, one spends about half the race cycling and the remaining half swimming and running. Your training should mimic this time distribution.

Another way to practice the principle of specificity is to simulate the topographical and climatic conditions of your next important race in the most useful ways possible in your training. For example, if you are training for a very hilly triathlon, you should incorporate plenty of hills into your bike and run training. Even little things like making sure to do at least some of your workouts at the same time of day as your approaching race or races can help you adapt more specifically to the demands of a race. With the same rationale, I recommend that you do some amount of your swim training in open water before any triathlon, instead of swimming only in pools.

Rule #3: Train Progressively

In order to stimulate an adaptation in any given system of your body, you must *overload* that system. In movies, the word "overload" is used only when something is about to explode. But in triathlon training, overload is your friend, as long as it's *progressive* in nature.

The principle of progressive overload is based on the fact that the body adapts best when it adapts gradually and consistently. A training effort represents an overload when it subjects a system of the body to a stimulus that is *slightly* unusual in type or, more often, degree. (Stimuli that are more than slightly unusual in type or degree will cause injury or illness.) If the specific training stimulus is repeated, and not only repeated but also progressively intensified, such that it remains always slightly unusual, the affected systems will progressively adapt until the limit of their adaptive potential is reached. Adaptations tend to be most rapid in the beginning (good news for beginners) and to slow gradually as this limit is approached.

How long you can continue to enhance particular training adaptations through progressive overload depends on a variety of factors, not the least of which is the particular adaptation in question. For example, generally an athlete can overload for endurance longer than he or she can overload for speed before a break is needed. The sum of the various adaptations we pursue through triathlon training is *peak fitness*. The collective experience of triathletes past and present has consistently shown that one cannot continue to gain fitness for more than a few to several months before hitting a peak. This doesn't mean you'll never get any faster than you are after your first six months of triathlon training. It just means you need to rest and then repeat the whole training process from the beginning in order to reach a higher fitness peak. In this regard people are a lot like plants. We cannot grow or bear fruit throughout the year. We are deeply enmeshed in the cycles that control everything in nature.

Among the great challenges of the sport of triathlon is timing one's fitness peaks to coincide with one's most important races. The two main variables you need to manipulate properly in order to peak at the right time are the length of your preparation period and the rate at which you overload your body during it. For the best results, you want to allow enough time to gain fitness as slowly as possible without stagnating, because fitness peaks tend to be highest when they are most gradually approached.

Rule #4: Train by Frequency, Intensity, and Duration

There are three main ways to overload your body in triathlon training: by increasing the frequency, the intensity, or the duration of workouts. Let's look at each of these variables independently.

Frequency

For optimal performance in triathlon, you should train as frequently as possible without interfering with your body's ability to recover adequately from each workout performed. Just how often this proves to be depends on a number of factors, the most important of which is how frequently you've been training recently. Abrupt increases in exercise frequency are risky. A second limiting factor with respect to frequency is the quality of one's recovery. A full-time professional triathlete whose recovery consists of mid-afternoon naps, casual meals, and reading trashy novels, plus eight and a half hours of sleep at night, will be able to handle greater exercise frequency than the amateur triathlete whose recovery consists of a stressful full-time job, raising three kids, hurried meals, and seven hours of sleep at night. (Sound familiar?)

A third factor that determines how much frequency is appropriate has to do with the nature of the workouts performed. The more you vary mode, duration, and intensity, the more frequently you will be able to train. For example, a well-conditioned triathlete might continue to recover from a hard track workout while performing a moderate-intensity swimming workout just hours later, because the second workout does not significantly challenge the systems of the body that were challenged most in the first workout.

Intensity

Intensity refers to the rate at which your body is *presently* converting energy into movement relative to your body's *maximum* capacity to do so in the modes of swimming, cycling, and running. Intensity is the most important training variable of all because it has the most direct relationship to the physical adaptations that result from training. Each level of intensity—and the gradations are infinite—imposes a very specific set of demands on the body, which result in specific physical adaptations that become more pronounced (up to a point) the more time you spend training at that particular level of intensity. Each workout you perform should emphasize one (or occasionally more than one) of the following

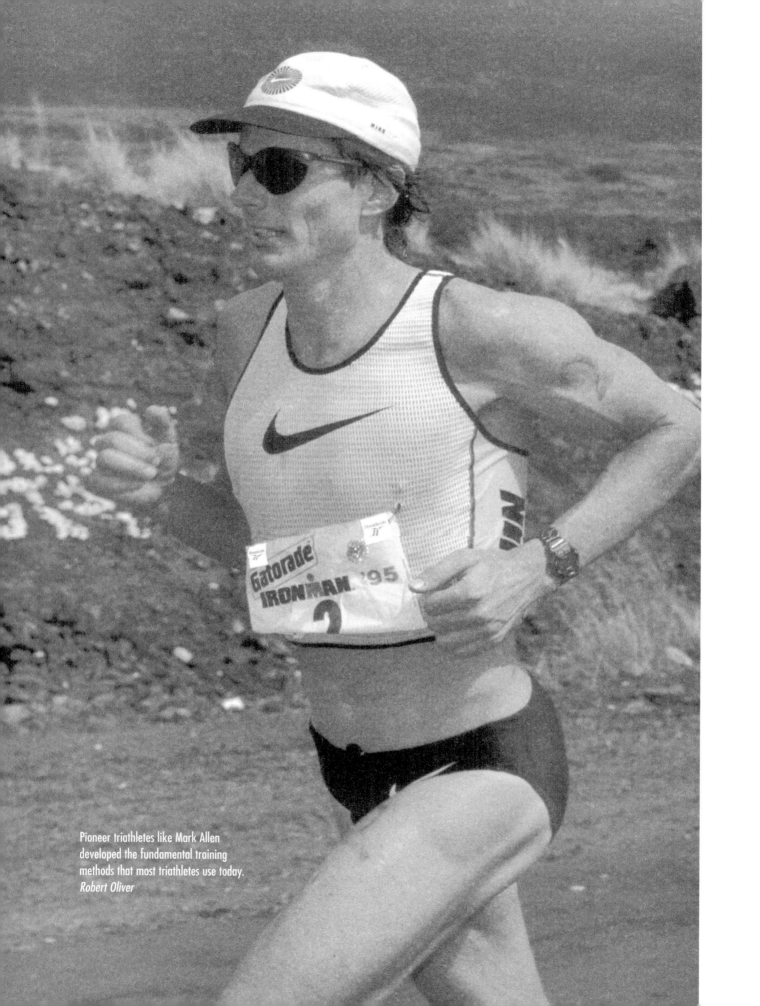

Pioneer triathletes like Mark Allen
developed the fundamental training
methods that most triathletes use today.
Robert Oliver

five intensities, for the sake of stimulating the specific adaptations associated with it:

1. Recovery

This is the lowest intensity of activity that still qualifies as exercise. In fact, well-conditioned triathletes achieve no fitness gains from training at this intensity level unless they really push the duration. The purpose of training at recovery intensity is not to increase fitness but instead to—you guessed it—*recover* from recent hard work by increasing circulation and flushing out metabolic wastes.

Recovery-intensity training is appropriate for warming up before workouts, cooling down after workouts, and engaging in active recovery between hard efforts within an interval type of workout, in which high-intensity efforts of relatively short duration are separated by low-intensity recovery periods, as well as for short workouts following races or particularly hard training sessions. For trained individuals, recovery intensity corresponds to roughly 55 to 65 percent of maximum rate of oxygen consumption (or *VO₂ max*) and 60 to 70 percent of maximum heart rate (*max HR*). Recovery pace feels very easy and only begins to feel hard as carbohydrate fuel becomes depleted after some time. For trained triathletes, maximum range at recovery pace is several hours. For beginners, there is no such thing as a recovery workout, because working out even at 60 percent of VO₂ max will increase aerobic fitness for such a person and therefore necessitate recovery rather than facilitate it. Beginners who need recovery should walk, stretch, or rest completely.

2. Endurance

The endurance intensity level is by far the most important training intensity for triathletes. If you were to use just one training intensity to prepare for a triathlon, this would be it. In fact, beginners should indeed train at this intensity level exclusively for a while (at least 12 weeks) before mixing in any of the higher intensities.

The endurance intensity level is really a broad intensity zone that lies between two physiological thresholds. On the low end, it is bordered by the threshold where fat burning peaks and carbohydrate burning overtakes fat as the primary fuel source. On the high end, it is bordered by the anaerobic threshold. Endurance workouts serve to increase oxygen consumption capacity and improve the body's ability to metabolize fat for fuel. Very long endurance workouts also improve carbohydrate storage capacity. In trained individuals, endurance intensity corresponds to roughly 65 to 75 percent of VO₂ max and 70 to 75 percent of max HR.

Endurance pace feels anywhere from easy to comfortable in the beginning and gradually becomes more challenging as carbohydrate fuel is depleted. For trained triathletes, maximum range at endurance pace is a few hours. Endurance workouts usually take the form of long (40 minutes to six hours), steady-pace swims, rides, and runs.

3. Threshold

The anaerobic threshold is the intensity level at which lactic acid suddenly begins to accumulate rapidly in the blood due to the body's inability to supply oxygen fast enough to break down all the fuel needed for energy, hastening exhaustion. Training at or near this intensity level is a very powerful means of improving oxygen consumption capacity, carbohydrate fuel-burning efficiency, and lactate clearance capacity, but only for those who have built a solid base of aerobic fitness through lower-intensity training.

Note that, unlike the recovery and endurance intensities, which represent general ranges, threshold intensity (as its name implies) is a very exact intensity level. Trained individuals will reach this threshold at a precise point somewhere between 80 to 90 percent of VO_2 max and 80 to 90 percent of max HR (depending on fitness level). Threshold pace feels comfortably hard initially and becomes gradually and steadily harder. For trained triathletes, maximum range at threshold pace is about an hour. Threshold workouts should take the form of sets of long intervals (for example: 3 x 12 minutes or 2 x 20 minutes) separated by active recoveries.

4. Max Oxygen

When you increase the intensity of swimming, biking, or running beyond the anaerobic threshold, you will soon reach another threshold, namely, VO_2 max, also called the ventilatory threshold, where your working muscles are taking up as much oxygen as possible. It is important, when engaging in max oxygen training, that you do not exceed the *minimum* intensity level at which VO_2 max is saturated, because doing so will decrease the amount of time you're able to spend at this intensity level and will therefore unnecessarily limit the desired training effects, which are to increase VO_2 max, carbohydrate burning efficiency, and lactate clearance capacity.

In trained individuals, max oxygen intensity corresponds to 95 to 100 percent of VO_2 max and 90 to 95 percent of max HR. Max oxygen pace feels hard initially and uncomfortable within just a few minutes. For trained triathletes, maximum range at max oxygen pace is about 15 minutes. Max oxygen workouts are typically performed in an interval format with hard efforts lasting three to five minutes.

5. Speed

Speed intensity usually corresponds to a pace that is 5 to 10 percent faster than threshold pace, but it can range up to a full sprint. Triathletes should use the speed intensity level sparingly, because it's highly stressful and quite a bit faster than race pace. Nevertheless, it serves three important functions for triathletes, and therefore should not be eschewed altogether. First of all, it improves your lactate clearance capacity by forcing you to work through acidosis (lactic acid accumulation) in a fairly high number of short, high-intensity intervals (e.g., 8 x 2 minutes @ 90 percent of maximum velocity). Second, it improves economy of movement, as technique tends to improve at higher speeds. And third, it limits the deterioration of raw speed that can accompany heavy endurance training.

In trained athletes, speed intensity corresponds to roughly 100 to 105 percent of VO_2 max and 95 to 100 percent of max HR. Speed pace feels very hard from the get-go. For trained triathletes, maximum range at speed pace is as little as 15 seconds for a full sprint and no more than about four minutes at a sub-sprint.

Methods of gauging and controlling intensity have been among the hottest training-related topics in the triathlon community in recent years. There are several such methods, which include the monitoring of pace, heart rate, blood lactate concentration, perceived exertion, and power output. My recommendation is that you rely on pace (that is, time over distance) as your primary gauge of intensity and supplement this by using perceived exertion and, if you wish, by using heart rate monitoring for cycling and running and perhaps power output as well for cycling. The rationale behind a pace-based approach is twofold. First, in triathlon we race by the clock, so why not train by it? Second, methods of endurance training have evolved very little since the days when athletes trained by pace exclusively. In other words, training by pace works, and it's also the simplest way of controlling intensity. Why complicate things unnecessarily? The workouts I will present in later chapters are all pace-based.

A Summary of the Five Training Intensities

The following table provides a summary of information about the five basic intensity levels used in triathlon training. Note that the "Feels Like" column refers to how each given intensity level feels initially. The longer you go at any intensity level, the harder it feels. The numbers in the "Percent of Total Training" column represent an average for the three training phases (discussed below) and for the three triathlon disciplines, whereas the actual numbers will need to vary by phase and by training mode. For example, in the base phase, at least 90 percent of your training should be performed at endurance intensity, and you'll always want to do more high-intensity training in swimming than you do in cycling and running. The "Maximum Range" column refers to how long a well-trained triathlete can maintain a given intensity level, not a beginner. Range, too, depends on mode. Most athletes can cycle much longer than they can run.

	Physiology	Feels Like	Training Effects	Percent of Total Training	Maximum Range
Recovery	Fat and carbohydrate burned in equal amounts	Very easy	Loosens and flushes metabolic wastes from muscles	10–15	10 hours +
Endurance	Carbohydrate burning predominates, but 100 percent of fuel burned aerobically (i.e., with oxygen)	Easy to slightly challenging	Increases oxygen consumption, fat burning, and carbohydrate storage capacities	70–80	6–10 hours
Threshold	Rate of carbohydrate burning begins to exceed rate of oxygen supply, lactic acid waste production spikes	Moderately hard	Increases oxygen consumption and carbohydrate-burning and lactate clearance capacities	8–12	60–90 minutes
Max Oxygen	Maximum rate of oxygen consumption is reached	Very hard	Increases oxygen consumption and carbohydrate-burning capacities and lactate clearance	3–5	15–20 minutes
Speed	Energy production is substantially or predominantly anaerobic, lactic acid accumulation is very rapid	Very hard to maximal	Increases efficiency and lactate clearance	2–3	1–5 minutes

Table 1.1

Duration

Duration, of course, has to do with how long a given workout lasts. The appropriate duration of each workout is determined by the intended effect of the workout, its intensity (which along with duration is a primary determinant of the workout's training effect), your present level of fitness, and the length of the race or races for which you are preparing.

While longer workouts are associated with greater gains in endurance and aerobic capacity, you most certainly do not want to make every workout last as long as possible. There are two reasons why this is the case. First, you will wind up overtrained and therefore less fit (if not injured) if you push the duration of workouts too often. Additionally, the longer your workouts last, the less intense they can be and the less frequently you can do them. As a triathlete you must always maintain a dynamic balance among the variables of duration, frequency, and intensity, because each of them carries benefits that the others do not. By doing one overdistance workout per week in each discipline, on average, you will reap all the benefits of pushing duration without having to cut back on intensity in other workouts or reduce overall workout frequency.

Closely related to duration is training *volume,* which is the total or average amount of time you spend training within a given period, usually a week or month. As with workout duration, the particular training volume that is appropriate for you at any given time depends on your recent training volume, the length of the peak triathlon you're preparing for, and where you are in the training cycle.

Your training *workload* is the total amount of energy you expend in training during a period of time—so it is a function of volume and intensity. Given two triathletes, each of whom trains 15 hours per week, the triathlete carrying the greater workload will be the one whose training has the higher average intensity. The particular training workload that is appropriate for you at any given time also depends on your recent training workload, the length of the peak triathlon you're preparing for, and where you are in the training cycle.

Rule #5: Train in Phases

For the best results, you should not work on all the important training adaptations throughout your entire training program. Put another way, you should not perform every type of workout every week. On the contrary, you will build a higher fitness peak by concentrating on different types of training at different times and sequencing these phases in a way that best allows each of them to build on the results of the preceding. The use of training phases is predicated on the following three discoveries made by earlier generations of triathletes and other endurance athletes:

1. You Need a Solid Foundation

Triathletes can handle a greater volume of training and more intense training if high volume and intensity are preceded by a period of strictly low-intensity training that increases in volume very gradually. First of all, such a buildup strengthens the bones, muscles, and connective tissues of the body, rendering them better able to handle the heavier and harder training to follow. Second, improving your aerobic capacity through sub-threshold training will help you get more out of high-intensity training later.

2. Your Training Should Get Increasingly Specific

The bulk of the training you do at actual race intensity should occur in the latter portion of the training process. This is the case for two reasons. First, race intensity is the intensity for which you want your body to be best adapted, and as an athlete, you are always best adapted to the type of training that has been your most recent focus. Second, in order to make race-intensity workouts really count, it's best if you're already in pretty good shape when you start doing them, so you can train longer at this intensity. Presumably, you're in better shape toward the end of the training cycle than toward the beginning.

3. You Need to Rest to Peak

Your heaviest training workload should fall in the middle portion of the training process. (Remember that workload is a function of training volume and intensity.) In other words, do the greatest amount of high-intensity training after you've built a solid foundation and before you begin to emphasize race-intensity workouts in the final phase of training. The reason you want your workload to peak well before you achieve an actual fitness peak for your most important race is that you'll be too tired to race well otherwise. In fact, the final week to three weeks of the training process should be the lightest of all.

In view of these three realities, dividing the training process into distinct phases is crucial. Individual training phases are not as abrupt or disparate as perhaps the term makes them sound. It's not like you do nothing but ride the bike in one phase and then quit cycling for two months in the next phase of training. Many elements of training remain constant and many patterns continue as one phase passes into the next. For example, in all three phases, the majority of your workouts should be steady-pace, endurance-intensity workouts. The main thing that does distinguish the training phases from one another is the types of workout that serve as *key* workouts in each.

The use of phases in sports training is commonly referred to as *periodization*. In triathlon there are several different systems of periodization with various numbers of phases and names for them. I prefer a simple, three-phase training cycle that includes a base phase, a build phase, and a peak phase. The *base phase* involves building a foundation of solid aerobic fitness by doing an increasingly heavy volume of low- to moderate-intensity swimming, biking, and running. This is also the time to enhance the body's capacity to handle heavy and hard training by increasing strength and flexibility and also to focus on technique improvement. In the *build phase,* you then push the limits of your aerobic fitness by doing as much high-intensity training as you can handle. In the *peak phase,* your goal is to maximize race-readiness through a combination of key workouts that stimulate the most race-specific adaptations and adequate rest. As your peak race approaches, the peak phase becomes a *taper,* a one- to three-week period of light training, which some coaches and athletes like to consider a separate, mini-phase.

Rule #6: Train in Cycles

Have I just contradicted myself? A moment ago I told you to train in phases. I've just now told you to train in cycles. Can one do both? Yes, one must!

A cycle is, of course, a pattern that recurs. Cycles are useful in triathlon training because they help organize the training process and also because certain patterns *must* recur in training if the program is going to result in progressively increasing fitness. You can't perform just one threshold-intensity workout and expect to thereby raise your anaerobic threshold, for example. I recommend the use of three levels of cycles: weekly cycles, step cycles, and full training cycles.

Weekly cycles are often referred to as micro-cycles. They are used not just because everybody in our society arranges most habitual activities in weekly cycles, but also for physiological reasons. Specifically, it just

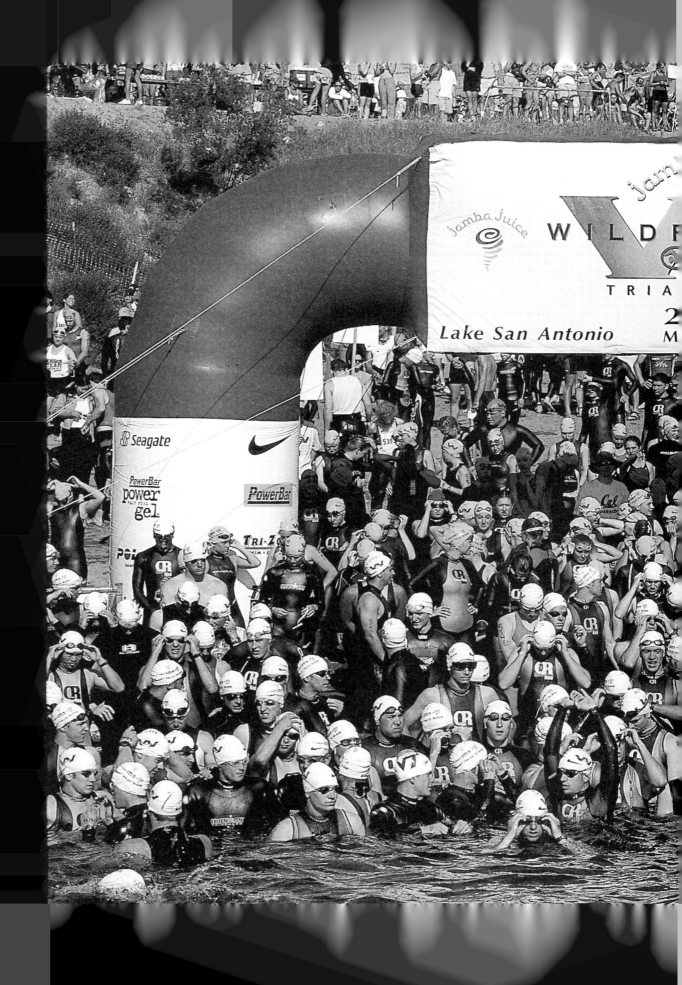

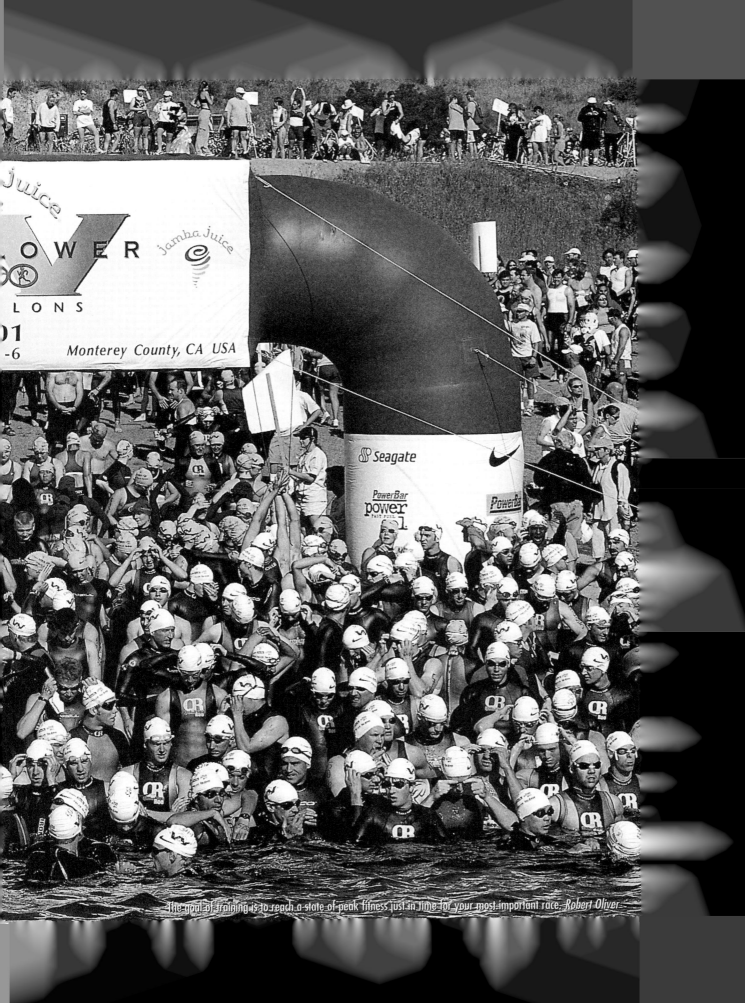

The goal of training is to reach a state of peak fitness just in time for your most important race. *Robert Oliver*

so happens that the training effect of a given workout type can be sustained only if the workout is repeated at least once a week (or so). Creating an optimal weekly training schedule is a game with two objectives. The first objective is fitting in all the necessary workouts; the second is arranging them in such a way that each specific stimulus is absorbed optimally, which typically entails surrounding each important workout with adequate rest and with workouts as unlike it (in mode, duration, and intensity) as possible. Most triathletes choose to do their heaviest training on the weekends, not for scientific reasons but rather for lifestyle ones.

Weekly cycles, in turn, are arranged into two- to four-week step cycles in which you repeat the basic pattern of a training week from one week to the next but increase the workload with each go-around, until the last week of the cycle, in which the workload is reduced for recovery. By incorporating planned recovery into your training program in this manner you can actually train harder during your hardest weeks and build more gradually toward a higher fitness peak than you could achieve if you tried to increase the workload every week. Each of the three training phases, base, build, and peak, should contain a certain number of complete step cycles; the precise number depends on the length of the overall training program.

Finally, the training program itself is a cycle in the context of your career as a triathlete. Most triathletes complete one *full training cycle* per year, but you can fit in two, or even three. Endurance is built over many years. Some of the physiological adaptations to training that increase endurance, such as the proliferation of cell mitochondria, can intensify continually from childhood until middle age. This puts veterans of high school track and swim teams at an advantage as adult triathletes, but it also means that those who come to triathlon as adults with no background in endurance sports can expect to make progress for several consecutive seasons just by staying consistent in their training. But this progress can only occur in cycles. You cannot actively pursue a fitness peak at all times of the year without breaking down eventually. Every triathlete needs an off-season.

Rule #7: Rest and Recover Sufficiently

As a training variable, rest denotes any time spent absorbing a recent training stimulus. Rest is the forum for recovery and adaptation. Except for improvements in neuromuscular coordination, all of the various physical adaptations that constitute increased fitness occur during rest rather than during workouts themselves. It is important never to lose sight of the fact that you cannot achieve optimal fitness without adequate rest.

Recovery and adaptation are more or less the same process. After a given system of the body has been overloaded, it must recover—that is, it must return to *homeostasis*—a state of balance or equilibrium. When a system of the body is overloaded habitually and progressively, it tends to go beyond homeostasis in the recovery process, and this constitutes adaptation. For example, a single workout will diminish carbohydrate stores, so that afterward the body must replenish them. A progressive sequence of workouts will result in the body's becoming gradually able to store more carbohydrate in the muscles, making it harder to deplete the supply. This process of adapting beyond homeostasis through the recovery process is called *supercompensation*.

Simply not exercising is not the only way to promote recovery. In fact, exercise itself can promote recovery in the right circumstances. By doing short, low-intensity workouts between longer, harder ones, you can accelerate the components of recovery that depend on circulation. It is also possible to fail to recover properly despite not exercising. Adequate sleep, proper nutrition, and stress management all have a profoundly beneficial impact on the recovery process. If you neglect to eat right, for example, no amount of rest will get you ready for your next hard workout. Your entire lifestyle is relevant to your progress as a triathlete.

Rest is tricky. While it is universally acknowledged that a higher level of performance is achievable only in a rested state, it is also understood that this moment of complete recovery is followed immediately by *detraining,* or the gradual loss of fitness, unless new stimulus is applied. In other words, no sooner have you fully adapted to your training than you begin to readapt to inactivity (in the absence of new training stimuli). The various physiological components of fitness deteriorate at different rates (for example, blood plasma volume is lost more slowly than capillary density)—but they all deteriorate sooner or later unless new challenges are absorbed. Consequently, successful training entails maintaining the right balance between the application of training stimuli and subsequent recovery. If you do not stress the right systems often or progressively, fitness gains will plateau and then reverse. If you skimp on recovery, however, you'll feel awful, and then get hurt or sick and feel even worse.

It is neither possible nor desirable to do every workout in a state of complete recovery from the previous one, however. This is due to the fact that, by forcing your body to work out a little more frequently than it wants to, you can train it to recover and adapt more quickly and to handle more work, which will lead to further fitness gains. This is why the variable of frequency is so important. I'll never forget how I felt when I first made the transition from working out once a day to working out twice a day several times a week. I gained fitness so quickly, it was almost dizzying.

The only times you need to achieve complete recovery are before important races and after a given training cycle ends. But this is not to suggest that you should take on a maximal workload at all other times. In order to even be able to handle a truly maximal workload during any given week you need to allow yourself a recovery week at least once a month—that is, you need to use step cycles. These recovery weeks are not as light as taper weeks, and therefore do not result in total recovery, but they come close enough to allow you to train harder when you train hard.

Rule #8: Customize and Evolve Your Training

Each triathlete is unique, and no two triathletes can achieve their best results through identical training programs. For this reason, it is essential that you customize your triathlon training to your particular needs and circumstances. There are two forms of customization: pre-adjustment and post-adjustment. Pre-adjustment entails planning your training in a more or less atypical way based on your personal exigencies. The most common reasons for pre-adjusting one's training away from the norm are schedule constraints and individual weaknesses. For example, a triathlete who's a strong cyclist and runner but a poor swimmer might choose to spend more than the typical 25 percent of his or her total training time practicing the swim until substantial improvement has been made.

Post-adjustment entails modifying your training based on the results of the training and racing you've done. The most common reasons for post-adjusting one's training are limitations or flaws perceived in previously used methods, injury, improvement (which can allow one to handle more or harder training), new ideas (either original or borrowed), and new goals. For example, you may perform badly on the hills in a race and come away determined to include more strength and hill training in your program training. (Or perhaps you'll just avoid hilly races from now on!)

There is tremendous opportunity for improvement in paying careful attention to cause and effect in your training and race performances, making informed deductions, and acting upon them. If your training remains the same year after year, then you are undoubtedly repeating mistakes that could be corrected with greater mindfulness, and are failing to make adjustments that would accommodate the changing needs and capabilities of your body. Consider it one of your chief goals as a triathlete to become your own coach. When you first begin in the sport, you can do no better than to follow general advice from authoritative resources such as coaches, experienced triathletes, and magazines. This will get you started. But once you have fully internalized the established principles and proven methods of training, and also seen how you respond when you apply and practice them in various ways, *you* become the most qualified expert to direct your own further development as a triathlete.

Sooner or later you'll have your own training philosophy. Individual training philosophies do not quarrel over the established principles and proven practices I've discussed in this chapter. Rather, each finds its own preferred spot within the field of possibilities defined by these rules. For example, some triathletes like to practice another kind of cycle that I did not get into here called *focus periods,* in which they emphasize one mode at a time in a recurring sequence, as when a swim-focus period is followed by a bike-focus period is followed by a run-focus period, and so on. This practice and other similar ones are not intrinsically better or worse than the alternatives—they just work better for some triathletes. A training philosophy is nothing more than what works best for the creator of that particular philosophy. The mark of a true veteran triathlete is an approach to training that's a little different from everyone else's approach, but has a reason behind every aspect of it.

Talking Shop

My friend Bernie is a "retired" amateur triathlete who used to be among the top age-groupers* in the state of Hawaii. Back in the late 1980s and early 1990s, Bernie did most of his training with a group of similarly dedicated triathletes on the Big Island. Naturally, when they worked out together, Bernie and his friends talked, and when they talked, like all triathlon training cliques past and present, in Hawaii and everywhere else, they talked triathlon more often than not.

Such endless shoptalk served several purposes. First, it provided a basis for their bond. "My girlfriend certainly didn't want to hear about bicycle aerodynamics, but my training friends did," Bernie recalls. Second, it provided validation that minimized the friends' insecurities about their individual training patterns, nutrition habits, and so forth. And third, it provided a learning forum for the friends, as none of them knew everything the others knew. "You could never get enough information," Bernie says. "We were all hungry for more knowledge, and it was always so exciting to come away with a new idea to try out—it gave you hope for improvement."

Accumulating and trading knowledge is one of the joys of being a triathlete. In general, learning, being knowledgeable, and teaching are sources of pleasure for everyone, and all the more so when the subject matter is close to one's heart. The sport of triathlon affords each athlete a chance to enjoy the pleasures associated with giving and receiving knowledge. You could never even hope to learn everything there is to know about triathlon if you devoted your entire life to it. That would entail learning all there is to know about human anatomy and physiology, the biomechanics of swimming, cycling, and running, the principles and methods of strength and flexibility training, nutrition and hydration, sports psychology, sports medicine, bicycles and components, the design and manufacture of running shoes, the history of the sport, fluid dynamics, and even Newtonian physics—and more.

The best ways to enjoy learning about any of these topics are to read and to ask questions of your training friends, who will appreciate the opportunity to play expert. Don't fret about how much you don't know, but instead just relish the discovery process. There's a special thrill to be had in successfully changing your first flat tire, or finally realizing why certain foods are good for you and others are not. Keep at it, and sooner or later you, too, will have the opportunity to play expert, and perhaps even to win one of the ferocious triathlon debates that occasionally erupt in training groups like Bernie's. "Oh, yes, we had our share of those!" he admits.

Speaking of debates, keep in mind that, as the expression goes, "A little knowledge is dangerous." Be skeptical, verify, and always place new information in its proper context, lest you accept and act upon false wisdom—of which there is plenty passed around in the realms of health and fitness—and see your performance suffer as a result. As a rule, make only small and gradual changes in your training and diet (tweak, don't overhaul), and do so only when you've heard the recommended change from two or more trusted sources—like me!

---

* Amateur triathletes refer to themselves as "age-groupers" because they compete in divisions defined by gender and age, such as "male 40–44."

CHAPTER 2

Getting Equipped

Several years into his storied career as a professional triathlete, German long-distance specialist Jürgen Zäck began to suffer from crippling lower back pain. As triathlon was not only his passion but also his livelihood, Zäck sampled every potential remedy he could find, from physical therapy to plain old rest, yet his condition continued to worsen until he was forced to contemplate retirement. But then, as a last resort, Zäck changed bikes, replacing his traditional, diamond-frame steed with a bike whose seat sat perched atop a suspended beam that absorbed more shock. Riding it, in combination with his other treatments, made all the difference. His back healed and he returned to top form.

The moral of this story is not that all triathletes should ride beam bikes, but simply that equipment matters. If you make the effort to choose and use the right stuff for you (and use it right), you will train more effectively, race faster, enjoy the sport more, and perhaps even enjoy it longer. Triathlon is a gear-intensive pursuit, which means that equipment represents an area of opportunity for triathletes who have the desire and wherewithal to take advantage of it.

Guidelines for Triathlon Shopping

Some triathletes consider shopping to be triathlon's unofficial fourth discipline. While it may not be quite *that* important, there's no question that making smart triathlon-related purchases can enhance your success in the sport. Savvy triathlon shopping is as simple as adhering to the following five guidelines:

1. Prioritize Purchases

Always prioritize essential purchases, such as shoe orthotics, supposing you need them to prevent injuries, ahead of all nonessential purchases. Always prioritize purchases that will enhance your enjoyment of the sport ahead of purchases you might feel you "ought" to make (perhaps because they are high priorities for your training partners). And as a general rule, purchase items that will help you train better ahead of those that will help you race better, and purchase items you will use frequently ahead of those you will use infrequently.

2. Purchase Equipment That Suits You

One good reason there are so many makes and models of bicycle is that there are so many different bodies. The same can be said of bike helmets, running shoes, and many other triathlon-related products. No single product in any of these categories is optimally suited to every triathlete. Swim goggles are a case in point. Goggles that fit your moon face perfectly are sure to leak or fog up on my pinhead. This may sound commonsensical, but many is the triathlete who buys products for no better reason than because they look good on a training partner, and regrets it.

The three keys to buying the right gear for you are, first, understanding the basic factors that differentiate products in any given category; second, understanding your equipment needs; and third, testing products prior to purchase whenever possible. The primary focus of the remaining sections of this chapter is to supply you with much of the information you'll need to make such informed buying decisions.

3. Pick a Good Retailer

The store you buy from matters almost as much as the products you buy, especially when the products are shoes and bikes, as the better retailers won't allow you to leave their stores with the wrong product. I'm talking about service. Many retailers that have just the right bike or shoe for you may not actually sell you that bike or shoe because of poor service—that is, because their personnel lack the knowledge or concern to match you up with it.

The hallmarks of a good retailer, beyond a great product selection, are personalized attention, knowledgeable salespeople who ask you lots of questions and offer well-considered answers to your own questions, and a policy of encouraging customers to test products. Stores with great service always carry a reputation for great service, which makes finding them easy if you ask around.

4. Use and Maintain Your Gear Properly

Your $200 heart rate monitor will never be worth more than 10 cents if you don't learn how to use the information it provides to refine your training. Likewise, buying a fancy triathlon bike will actually slow you down rather than speed you up if you never bother to properly fit it to you (or have your retailer do so). While many triathlon products are "wash-and-wear," others require an investment of care and attention to yield the full measure of their potential benefits. This is especially true in relation to your bike, which requires almost as much care and attention as a horse for optimal performance. I'll discuss basic bicycle maintenance and upkeep in Chapter 4.

5. Explore New Options

A triathlete's shopping is never done—at least, it shouldn't be. By this I mean that you'll be well served to remain always on the lookout for products that can enhance your enjoyment of, or performance in, triathlon, be it a product of a kind you've never tried before, a simple upgrade, or a new technology or recent invention.

Gearing Up for Triathlon

Let's now take a product-by-product look at the most essential and useful items of triathlon equipment and the most important factors to consider when shopping for and using them. This is not an exhaustive list, by any means. For example, not one word about hypoxic sleeping chambers!

Essential Swim Stuff

Swimsuit

Fit, hydrodynamics, and look are generally the virtues triathletes look for in swimsuits. Men may choose from among a wide variety of briefs, which leave little to the imagination; jammers, which are cut more like cycling shorts; and skin suits, which cover even more of the body with materials that reduce water drag and muscle vibration (which, apparently, slows down swimmers a tiny, tiny amount). Women have one-

Tips for the Budget Triathlete

If you give maybe 5 percent more effort in your triathlon shopping by bargain hunting, you'll spend perhaps 20 percent less money. Here are just five among dozens of ways to keep your triathlon spending from getting out of hand:

1. Buy "last year's" bike. Just like auto dealers, bike retailers offer big (10 to 20 percent) model-year-end discounts on brand-new bikes beginning in midsummer, when they need to make room for the next model year's inventory. You can score similar seasonal discounts by purchasing summer training apparel in the fall and winter apparel in the spring.

2. Buy sports nutrition in bulk. Triathletes can easily spend several hundred dollars a year on energy bars and drinks. You can get worthwhile volume discounts on this stuff when you buy in bulk from online and mail order discounters like endurancezone.com.

3. Join a club. Members of many local running, cycling, and triathlon clubs receive discounts when they shop from particular local retailers. Also, some stores and mail order companies sponsor savings clubs that encourage customer loyalty through discounts.

4. Buy used bike stuff. The eagerness of so many cyclists and triathletes to upgrade generates a large secondhand market and a great opportunity for multisport bargain hunters, especially given the durability of today's better frames and parts. Resources for used bike stuff include bike shops (for complete bikes only), cycling and triathlon clubs, health club bulletin boards, newsletters and newspapers, and various online news groups and Web sites. Try to avoid buying anything you can't inspect first.

5. Hit the expos. At triathlon expos, multisport product retailers generally sell their wares at big discounts off their regular store prices. To avoid impulse buying at these events, hit the next expo with specific needs in mind, even if you're not racing the next day!

piece, two-piece, and skin suit options to consider. Go for a fit that's snug but not constricting. Beyond material and body coverage, snugness of fit affects the suit's hydrodynamic properties most.

Never compete in triathlons using a traditional swimsuit. They are not designed to give you the protection you need on the bike. Instead, you'll need to wear a triathlon suit, which is basically a swimsuit–cycling short hybrid (see detailed description below). Also, I recommend that you own and use at least two swimsuits in training, so you always have one to wear while you're washing the other.

Goggles

By far the most important consideration with goggles is fit. Ill-fitting goggles can be uncomfortable and can leak. Factors affecting fit are lens shape, gasket design (the gasket is the part of the goggle that touches your face), and strap design. Never buy a pair of goggles without first trying it on—and even this measure is not foolproof. Goggles that feel great will sometimes leak, too. Fortunately, most goggles are cheap, so you can always try, try again if necessary without taking a major hit in the wallet. A goggle alternative for those who find all goggles uncomfortable is swim masks designed for fitness swimming rather than diving.

The second most important consideration with goggles is visibility. Special visibility features in some goggles include tinted lenses for outdoor use, anti-fog lenses, or even corrective lenses for the nearsighted. Frankly, I have rarely found so-called anti-fog lenses that perform as they're promoted to do. To make your lenses truly fog-free, pick up a bottle of anti-fog solution from your performance swimwear or multisport retailer and simply spread a small drop around the inside of the lenses before each use. (Baby shampoo also works.)

Useful Swim Stuff

Triathlon Suit

Triathlon suits—tri-suits—are technical garments designed specifically for triathlon racing. While I mention them here among swim gear, they are worn through all three legs of the triathlon (often underneath a wetsuit in the swim). Made in one- and two-piece varieties for men and women, they combine a swimsuit's sleekness, the seat-area protection (and sometimes the thigh compression) of a cycling short, and the torso coverage of a cycling jersey or running top. There's a great deal of variety in triathlon suit designs. For example, among two-piece designs, you can choose tops with and without sleeves, with and without a rear pocket, with and without a front zipper, and in full-length or short-cut (or sports bra) varieties, to say nothing of the various fabric types available.

Although triathlon suit design preferences are highly individual, typically, suits that feature greater seat protection and thigh compression are preferred for longer triathlons, while sleekness and lightness (less fabric) are preferred for shorter events.

Wetsuit

Triathlon wetsuits were created in order to keep triathletes warm in cold water, but they also make triathletes more buoyant, hence faster, in open water, once you've adjusted to the different feel of swimming in one. Perhaps knowing that it serves two purposes will make you feel better about shelling out for a wetsuit, as you can expect to pay at least $300 for a full suit. However, as with a good bike frame, a good wetsuit will last a whole career if you take proper care of it (rinse and air-dry it after each use and store it inside out).

Factors to consider when choosing a wetsuit are fit, ease of motion (in the shoulders especially, for full suits), and ease of removal, as the faster you can get the damn thing off, the faster your first transition will be. Triathlon wetsuits come in full suit, half suit, sleeveless, and two-piece varieties. Most models feature variable-thickness neoprene construction (thicker in the legs for buoyancy) and a long zipper in back.

Swim Cap

Swim caps reduce drag, protect hair from chlorine and salt, and improve visibility for those with longer hair. If you do have longer hair, consider the swim cap an essential piece of equipment; otherwise, it's optional. The cheapest swim caps are made of tight-fitting latex and differ from one another only in appearance. Most triathlon events distribute color-coded latex swim caps to distinguish the several starting waves. Keep these and you may never have to buy one! Silicone caps tend to be a little more comfortable (less hair pulling) and a little more expensive. Lycra fabric swim caps are even more comfortable but are also less sleek in the water.

Swim Aids

Included in this category are swim fins, paddles, pull buoys, and kickboards. I will discuss these items in the next chapter when I talk about the training drills for which they're used.

Essential Bike Stuff

Bike

The bike is your most important triathlon purchase by a long shot. I say this not just because the bike is the costliest purchase you'll make (unless you buy and install a pool or something), but also because it is the item of equipment that has the greatest impact on your race times, and because there are more choices available in this product category than in any other, and because choosing the bike that's best suited to you requires more care than is the case with any other equipment item.

Finding the right bike is more challenging the less experience you have as a cyclist. This is because finding the right bike is primarily a matter of feel—of how the riding experience on one bike compares against your encounters with other bikes, and the more experienced rider is better attuned to the nuances of the riding experience. Nevertheless, for new and veteran cyclists alike, proper bike-shopping methodology is the same: after limiting your search by deciding how you intend to use your bike (hence what type of bike you need) and how much dough you can afford to spend on it, you must thoroughly test several bikes and purchase the bike that *feels* best, keeping in mind the intended application.

Expect to pay at least $1,000 for a road bike that is race-worthy and at least $1,200 for an entry-level triathlon bike. Expect to find that more expensive bikes generally perform better. If you lack that kind of scratch, you'll need to simply save up or else buy used, but even then, pay attention to more than just the price. Thoroughly inspect any used bike you consider buying for wear (especially frame cracks), or have a bike expert do so on your behalf, and bear in mind that it's rarely worth buying a fixer-upper. Between the bike itself and the needed upgrades, you'll probably wind up spending more than you would have dished out for a new bike of equal quality.

When shopping for a new bike, never assume that what you see is what you must get. If you like everything about a bike you're considering except the seatpost, for example, tell your salesperson you don't like the seatpost and see what he or she can do about it. Any reasonable shop will give you fair trade-in value for substitutions. For that matter, in keeping with shopping principle number five discussed above, it's always wise to consider your bike a work in progress, even years after you've brought it home. At any given time, there's probably at least one fit-, comfort- or performance-enhancing adjustment or upgrade you can make, even if it's changing your handlebar tape or choice of chain lubricant.

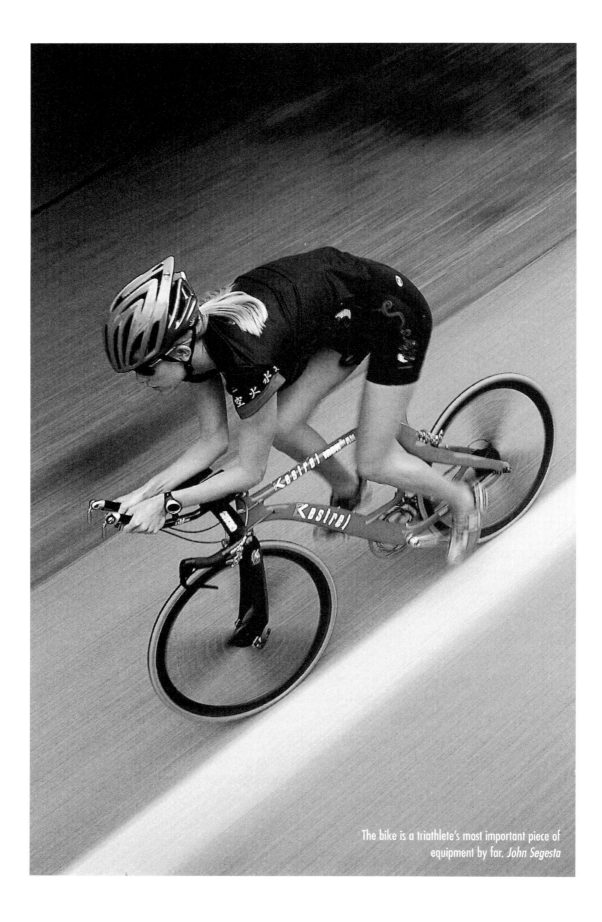

The bike is a triathlete's most important piece of
equipment by far. *John Segesta*

After you've established your budget, your next consideration is whether to buy a triathlon bike or a road bike, or both. This consideration is your second way of limiting your bike search before engaging in test rides and is based on your experience level, body proportions and pedaling biomechanics, and intended use for the bike. The essential difference between triathlon and road bikes is that triathlon bikes are designed to perform best in time trial conditions (flat and straight), whereas road bikes are designed to perform best on hills and turns and in pack riding. To serve their function, triathlon bikes position the rider differently than road bikes. Specifically, they tilt the rider forward several degrees more and place his or her forearms on an aerobar (except when cornering, breaking, climbing, relaxing, and sometimes shifting) for a low, stretched-out, and narrow riding position that maximizes aerodynamic efficiency. In order to make this position (reasonably) comfortable, tri-bikes use a shorter top tube, and in order to accommodate the more forward distribution of the rider's weight, they often have a tighter wheelbase. Further, to make the tighter wheelbase feasible, triathlon bikes sometimes come equipped with smaller wheels.

The aero position afforded by the triathlon bike's design offers a tremendous advantage in terms of efficiency in time trial conditions. It requires far less power output for the rider to maintain any given speed in the aero position in such conditions than it does when he or she pedals in the various road cycling positions. Given this fact, you may wonder why anyone would use anything other than a triathlon bike for triathlon training and racing. Two reasons. First, the aero position is really a racing position. While fast, it's not as comfortable or stable as the road positions. Nor do triathlon bikes perform as well as road bikes when ridden in any other position (hands on brake hoods, for instance) or on hilly terrain. For these reasons, most triathletes who have two bikes do most of their training on a more versatile road bike. Second, it's fairly easy to modify a road bike to accommodate an aero position that's nearly as efficient as that of a tri-bike. You just need to buy a clip-on aerobar and perhaps a forward seatpost, and then fine-tune a bit. In fact, even some professional triathletes (usually tall men with longer torsos) race on modified road bikes in long-distance events, where comfort and versatility are more important.

So, who should get which kind of bike? A triathlon bike is seldom a good option as a first bike for the relatively inexperienced cyclist. It's generally better to get a road bike and a clip-on aerobar (and a forward seatpost, if need be) and ease into aero riding in this way. If race times matter to you more than versatility and comfort in training, and if you do mostly shorter triathlons, and if you can't afford two bikes just yet, then, and only then, it may be worth getting a triathlon bike first. In any case, the ideal scenario is to own two bikes, of course, unless you do mostly long-distance triathlons and your body proportions are such that you are able to find a very efficient aero position on a road bike, in which case a triathlon bike may be superfluous.

This leads us to the matter of feel, which has three interrelated components: fit, comfort, and performance. Fit is all about achieving a riding position that balances aerodynamics and power production. This optimal riding position, in turn, is a function of frame size, bike proportions, and final adjustments, or fitting. Again, the various road bike positions (there are several possible hand placements on a road handlebar) tend to be more powerful (and more comfortable), while the triathlon bike's aero position is more aerodynamic. Road and triathlon bike frames are sized by the measurement of their top tube length, in centimeters. However, each manufacturer chooses its own precise endpoints for the measurements, such that it's not uncommon for a 56-centimeter frame of Brand X to actually have a 55-centimeter top tube, while a 56-centimeter frame of Brand Y actually has a 57-centimeter top tube. Consequently, cyclists never have a single, invariant bike size, like a pant size, but rather a *size range*. So, to find a good fit, the thing to do is mount a bike that's in your size range and rotate the right pedal down to the bottom of its cycle. Without angling your hip, extend your right leg and try to place your heel on the pedal. If you can just barely do it (in shoes), without adjusting the seat stem to the very top or bottom of its range, the frame is approximately the right size.

However, it still may not be the right bike for you on account of the proportions factor. Two bikes with identical top tube measurements might have different drop tube lengths, different geometry, different crank lengths, different front stem sizes, and so forth. At the same time, two riders with identical torso lengths might have different inseams, arm lengths, foot lengths, weight measurements, pedaling biomechanics, and so on. All of these measurements and proportions play a role in fit. Does this mean you have to take a bunch of measurements to find a good fit? No, because they all add up to something you can simply feel when riding: a good fit or a poor one.

Finally, it's rare that even the best-fitting bike among those you try will be adjusted exactly the way you need it on the showroom floor of the bike shop. This is where setup comes in—that is, fine-tuning saddle height and position, aerobar setup, and so forth. I'll discuss setup in Chapter 4.

If comfort were the most important quality of a racing bike, triathletes would race on massive cruisers with fat, cushy seats, big, soft tires, and slack geometry. But because *speed* is the most important quality of a racing bike, and because speed and comfort tend to work at cross-purposes, racing bikes are never super-comfortable. However, if a bike is less than reasonably comfortable, speed will suffer, especially over longer distances. So, what you want is a racing bike that feels very comfortable—for a racing bike.

The factor that most affects comfort is, again, fit. If your bike is the right size and your riding position is correct, you will be about as comfortable as you can be on a racing bike. That said, frame stiffness and design also make a difference. Less stiff frames tend to absorb more shock and therefore feel more comfortable. As for design, shock-absorbing beam bikes like the one Jürgen Zäck switched to are very popular among triathletes, many of whom feel that this design leaves their legs less beat-up for the run.

The saddle also affects comfort, for obvious reasons. Some saddles offer more padding and support than others, but these tend to weigh more and are sometimes bulky. If you can learn to live with a bony, ultralight racing saddle, do so; otherwise, a compromise measure that works well for many cyclists is placing a padded seat cover over the racing saddle. Note that, regardless of your saddle type, bike fit, and frame material, if you're new to cycling, you can expect to feel some normal discomfort in your seat area, neck, lower back, and perhaps also in your hands and other areas; this discomfort will diminish as your body adjusts to riding.

The performance component of bike feel has to do with how well a given bike moves in various circumstances (climbing, cornering, etc.), which is a function primarily of weight, stiffness, aerodynamics, and components. A lighter bike accelerates more quickly, often handles more nimbly, and performs much better on hills. Weight is affected most by materials. Of the four major frame materials, carbon fiber is lightest, followed by titanium, aluminum, and steel. Lightness is also a virtue of better bike components. To upgrade bike parts is generally synonymous with replacing heavier parts (aluminum front fork, aluminum seatpost) with lighter ones (carbon fiber front fork, titanium seatpost). As a general rule, you should get the lightest bike and components possible without giving up aerodynamics, fit, or too much comfort or durability.

Bike stiffness is determined mainly by the composition and design of the frame. Stiffness is considered a factor in bike performance because a stiffer bike dissipates less energy, especially when climbing, and handles better, especially at high speeds and when cornering. Generally, carbon fiber is the stiffest material, followed by steel, titanium, and aluminum, but because design is also an important factor, it is possible for an adroitly built aluminum bike to be stiffer than certain carbon fiber ones. It is easy to compare the relative stiffness of various bikes just by riding them. Riders often describe the feel of a bike that lacks sufficient stiffness as "squirrelly." However, the degree of stiffness that feels best to any given cyclist is an individual matter, as stiffer bikes (again) offer less shock absorption, which can compromise comfort.

Aerodynamics are affected most of all by rider position, which (you guessed it) has to do with fit. With tri-bikes and modified road bikes, the goal is to achieve the most stretched-out and streamlined aero position possible without any significant sacrifice in comfort or the amount of power you're able to generate (and one does tend to lose power as one gains in aerodynamics). When testing road bikes without aerobars, pay attention to power production more than aerodynamics, as there's little advantage to be gained in the latter.

The actual shape of the frame has a smaller effect on drag than rider position, but a significant effect still. More or less, the narrower the profile of the frame, the more aerodynamic it is. So-called aero frames are easily identified by their bladelike bottom and drop tubes. After the frame, wheels have the next biggest impact on aerodynamics. So-called aero wheels are easily identified by their wide, deep-dish rims and their low spoke count. Closely related to the factor of aerodynamics is that of rolling resistance, which refers to the amount of energy that is lost as heat where the rubber meets the road. Factors that affect rolling resistance are tire width (the lesser the better), tire pressure (the higher the better), and bike-rider weight (the lower the better).

The final component of bike performance is, well, components—that is, the bike's mechanical components: shift levers, brake levers, brakes, cables, derailleurs, freewheel, chainrings, chain, sprockets, crankset, and hubs. To understand why these parts are important you need consider nothing more than the fact that, without them, the bike could neither move nor stop. Two companies dominate the market for component groups, as they're called: Shimano and Campagnolo. Almost any high-quality triathlon or road bike you buy today will come equipped with Shimano 105, Dura-Ace, or Ultegra components, or a mix thereof, or Campagnolo Daytona, Chorus, or Record components, or a mix thereof. Even the worst of these components are just plain fantastic as compared to the components of a decade ago. They're light, precise, and durable. Yes, the most expensive groups are fractionally lighter, more precise, and more durable than the less expensive ones, so there is reason to upgrade, but if your bike is equipped with any of the above-mentioned component types, I would prioritize other upgrades first. On the other hand, if you should buy a nice fifteen-year-old frame with a fifteen-year-old component group, I would upgrade the component group first.

Helmet

Helmets are mandatory in all triathlons and should be considered mandatory for every ride. All helmets used in USAT (USA Triathlon)–sanctioned triathlons must also be ANSI (American National Standards Institute)– and Snell-certified (virtually every bike helmet on the market is thus certified). The ideal helmet will fit snugly, offer plenty of ventilation, be very light and aerodynamic—and match your bike! Costlier performance helmets tend to be substantially superior to cheaper helmets in terms of aerodynamics, ventilation, and weight. Pay attention to the comfort of the chin strap and ease of strap adjustment, buckling and unbuckling before buying.

Sunglasses

Performance sunglasses protect the eyes from three things: flying debris and insects, blinding sun glare, and ultraviolet radiation. Appropriate sunglasses for cycling will have full UV protection, shatterproof lenses, and excellent visibility; they'll also be very light and comfortable and won't slip despite sweat and the slightly downward-looking head position you maintain while riding. Some models offer interchangeable lenses so you can select the right lens color for current conditions.

Shoes and Pedals

Since 1984, flat pedals with toe clips have been obsolete. All competitive riders now use one or the other of the two main types of clipless pedal (Speedplay-compatible and LOOK-compatible), which are designed such that the cycling shoe locks right into them, allowing the rider to generate leverage more evenly throughout the pedal stroke. If you've never used clipless pedals, switch now. It's an easy adjustment and the advantage gained is big. Large-platform pedals are sometimes more comfortable and easier to lock into, while small-platform pedals are lighter. Cyclists with fickle knees often prefer pedals that allow some heel float, while other riders like the precise feel of pedals that allow no lateral movement. Note that most high-performance road and triathlon bikes do not come with pedals, so you should factor their cost into your bike budget if you don't have a pair already.

As for shoes, go for a snug, comfortable fit with a little room for foot swelling during long rides. The sole should be extremely rigid to minimize energy loss, although some riders prefer a little flexibility, especially when going long. A leather upper tends to be more comfortable than the plastic upper found in some of the less expensive shoes. Some shoes also offer better ventilation than others. A couple of bike shoe companies make triathlon-specific shoes that are easier to remove as you fly into transition.

Socks

Use socks that are designed for multisport use: that is, thin, low-cut socks made of moisture-wicking material that also protects against blisters.

Shorts

A good cycling short, or chamois (pronounced *shammy*), offers excellent seat-area padding and comfortable thigh support and is made of durable Nylon/polyester/spandex fabric that will last a career. More expensive shorts tend to be more durable and more comfortable (on the bike, not necessarily off it) than cheaper shorts. Never wear your chamois more than once without laundering it! That's a recipe for saddle sores, a painful condition that afflicts the perineum when sores caused by seat friction get infected.

Jersey

Your cycling jersey should fit fairly snugly to minimize wind drag and should feature breathable, moisture-wicking fabric to keep you cool. Individual styles differ from one another in fabric weight and feel as well as in collar, zipper, cuff, and pocket construction. The rest is fashion.

Hydration Systems

There are four ways to go with bicycle hydration systems. Water bottle cages attached to the drop and/or bottom tubes and designed to hold 16- to 28-ounce plastic water bottles are most commonly used in training. Many cyclists and triathletes prefer a cage that suspends one or two water bottles behind the seat, or a special hydration bladder with straw that is placed between the aerobars and allows the rider to drink hands-free, especially for racing. It's a matter of personal preference.

A fourth option is to wear a fluid bladder on your back (such as those made by CamelBak) and drink from a long tube that snakes out from it. These are most useful for very long rides in which you'll consume a lot

Upgrade and Save

Racing with excellent fitness and mediocre equipment is like building an
impregnable fortress and then defending it with the front door wide open.
If you want your race splits to be as low as possible, you'll want to not only
train for maximum fitness but also use the fastest available equipment.
Following are several categories of equipment upgrade and the approximate
time savings they can afford in the swim, bike, and run portions of an
Olympic-distance triathlon (1.5K/40K/10K).

The Swim

Upgrade	Time Savings
No wetsuit to wetsuit	1:30

This figure is an extrapolation based on testing performed in a pool environment by kinesiologists at the University of Calgary, Canada.

The Bike

Upgrade	Time Savings
No aerobar to aerobar	3:24–4:36
Standard wheels to aero wheels	0:40–0:55
Shaving two kilos	0:05–1:12

These estimates were generated using a computer program created by Tom
Compton of Analytic Cycling. They assume a rider of average size and able to
generate a steady 250 watts of power on two separate courses, one flat, the
other hilly (hence the ranges in time savings). Note that, for the aerobar and
aero wheel upgrades, the greater time savings come on the flat course, while
for the weight-shaving upgrade (which can be achieved in a number of ways,
including rider weight loss!), the greater time savings come on the hilly course.

The Run

Upgrade	Time Savings
Training shoes to racing flats	0:30

This estimate is based on a formula created by E. C. Frederick, Ph.D., of Exeter
Research. Through testing, Frederick determined that distance runners gain 1 percent in performance for every 100 grams shaved off their shoes. Assumed here are
an athlete capable of a 45-minute 10K split (in trainers) and a weight reduction of
200 grams (which is easily achieved in replacing typical trainers with racing flats).

of fluid, but be advised that, when full, they add to the strain that cycling places on the lower back. Such bladders are also illegal in most triathlons.

Maintenance Stuff

This category includes chain lubricant, spare tubes and a patch kit, a hex wrench set for adjustments, carbon dioxide cartridges or a portable air pump (for on-the-road tire inflation), a floor pump, and cleaning solvent. Never ride without the materials you need to repair and/or replace punctured tubes or tires stowed in a saddle pouch underneath the back of your seat. Keeping your drive train clean and lubricated and your tires properly inflated is essential for performance.

Useful Bike Stuff

Race Wheels

After the frame, the bike parts on which you can save the most weight and gain the greatest aerodynamic advantage are wheels. The only problem is that you can expect to pay at least a grand to upgrade from stock wheels to race wheels. Also, be aware that durability can be an issue with the lightest wheels, especially for heavier riders.

Because top-end wheels are very expensive and typically less durable than less expensive wheels, many triathletes like to use separate wheel sets for training and racing. Note that many aero wheels are inefficient in crosswind conditions, for which reason you'll either want to have *two* sets of race wheels (a deep-dish set and a thin-rimmed set) or else use your training wheels on windy race mornings.

Many triathletes save a few additional ounces on wheels by riding on the smaller of the two common wheel sizes, 650c versus 700c (the "c" stands for millimeters, believe it or not). If you stand less than five feet ten or so, this is an option. If you're under five feet six or so, you *should* use 650c wheels. If you're about six feet or taller, you'll definitely feel more comfortable on the larger wheels.

Aerobar

There are two basic types of aerobar: the integrated aerobar that comes with any triathlon bike and the clip-on aerobar that attaches to a traditional road bike handlebar with a few turns of the screw. While integrated aerobar designs tend to be fairly similar, there are many very different designs of clip-on bar, so if you're riding a modified road bike, shop around before choosing one, as the wrong one could screw up your entire bike fit.

The other big choice to be made is between bar-end shifters, which allow you to shift (but not brake) without removing your hands from the aerobar, and integrated brake-shifter levers, which are located on the wings of your aerobar setup or on the drop area of your road bike handlebar. Bar-end shifters are generally preferred for flatter rides on which less shifting is required and can become a nuisance on hilly and twisty terrain. Purchasing both types of shifter and switching them when necessary offers the greatest versatility.

Gloves

Cycling gloves protect your hands from soreness and blistering on long rides. Be careful to choose gloves that won't cause you to overheat but are not so flimsy that they begin to come apart after three rides, as did a pair I once had.

Foul-Weather Clothes

This category includes long-sleeve jerseys, wind vests, jackets, ear warmers, tights, and foul-weather gloves. The better stuff is light, thin, form-fitting, breathable, and effectively fights the elements. Jackets and vests should be bright for visibility. Dressing right for cold and wet weather is an art form—most novices tend to overdo it. The worst mistake you can make is to wear cotton sweat clothes and other clothes that aren't designed specifically for cycling.

Bike Computer

A bike computer, or cyclometer, allows you to track information such as distance traveled, time elapsed, and average speed on a real-time basis as you ride. The fancier ones also monitor pedaling cadence and even power output. I highly recommend their use for competitive triathletes, as the information they provide is very useful for structuring workouts and for gauging fitness and performance.

Indoor Cycling Equipment

There are three main reasons to cycle indoors: to avoid bad weather, to train in a controlled environment, and to train by power output. There are a few different ways to ride inside. Wind trainers and rollers allow you to pedal in place using the bike you have. The main difference between the two devices is that rollers require balance. A side benefit of rollers is that they're useful in revealing pedal stroke inconsistencies. Wind trainers are generally preferable for longer indoor rides. The other option is a stationary bike designed for indoor use. If you take this route, I recommend using the models that function most like regular outdoor bikes, such as those used in indoor cycling classes. A special kind of stationary bike, called a bike ergometer, allows you to train by power output, which is the most absolute measurement of cycling performance.

Bike Rack/Bike Case

Unless you plan to ride your bike from home every time you ride it, you'll need a bike rack for your car. The options are trunk-mounted racks, roof-mounted racks, and interior racks (for vans and SUVs). Look for sturdiness and ease of operation when shopping.

And if you're going to travel to events by plane, you'll need a bike case. There are various designs: some tougher than others, some lighter than others, and so on. Note that all bike cases require bike disassembly and reassembly —but that's a good skill to learn anyway.

Essential Run Stuff

Running Shoes

Running shoes are your second most important purchase after the bike, mainly because nothing can do more to screw up your training and racing than the wrong shoe. The primary function of running shoes is to protect the feet and legs from injury while minimizing the speed loss that comes with confining and weighing down your bare foot.

When shopping for running shoes, avoid stores that sell any other kind of shoe. Buy only from running specialty stores whose sales personnel are runners, unless you go the mail order route, in which case you'd better know exactly what you're getting. When you find a shoe you like, stick with it (which, admittedly, is easier to advise than do, given how frequently shoe models are changed and discontinued). Too many runners start over every time they buy a new pair of running shoes, primarily because they allow their search to be led by salespeople who never bother to ask them what they're wearing currently and how it's working for them. Also, keep track of the mileage your shoes accumulate and the wear they show. A well-built trainer should perform well for 500 miles or so.

As with bikes, shop for shoes by feel, paying attention to the following factors: fit, comfort, stability, cushioning, and weight. And as with bikes, fit is clearly the most important consideration. The shoe's upper should hug your foot without constricting it and leave just enough toe room so that your toes don't jam into the front of the shoe when you run downhill. Be wary of partially good fits, such as shoes that hug the mid-foot nicely but slip in the heel. If your foot is unusually narrow or wide, learn which models come in special narrow-width or extra-wide varieties and go straight to these when shopping. Pay attention to the arch as well. If it feels like a lump of any sort, that's a sure sign that it doesn't match the contour of your own arch.

This leads us to comfort, which is largely just the feel of a good fit. A poor fit simply won't feel right, even if it's in one small part of the shoe. Don't assume that you could get used to such small flaws. Like those annoying little quirks we try to overlook in attractive new dates, these flaws are sure to become downright unbearable over time. Learn to listen to your feet.

Comfort also relates to cushioning and lateral motion. If a shoe's cushioning is too meager or too stiff, or if you feel your ankles roll inward in it, this won't feel comfortable either. Naturally, you'll more likely discover comfort flaws in a shoe when you actually run in it than when you're just standing in the store and looking down at it like a dork, so be sure and take a lap around the parking lot in any shoe you're considering buying.

Cushioning is the main duty of any running shoe, yet running shoes more often provide too much cushioning rather than too little. Excessive cushioning not only adds weight to the shoe but also exacerbates energy dissipation and lateral motion tendencies. My recommendation is that you go with as little cushioning as you can get away with, but try not to find out the hard way how little you can get away with. A cautious way to proceed is to replace each worn pair of running shoes with a slightly lighter pair until you've worked your way down to a nice lightweight trainer. This recommendation applies to wispy and hefty runners alike. Among the most prevalent running shoe myths is that heavier runners need the most cushioning. Actually, speed affects impact force far more than weight, and you don't see many elite marathoners training in fluffy marshmallow shoes, do you? If you have a predisposition for shin splints or other impact-related injuries, avoiding asphalt in favor of packed dirt will make a far greater difference than extra shoe cushioning. That said, if you currently run on fluffy marshmallow shoes and like 'em just fine, more power to you.

Most running shoes offer stability features to make up for the instability that is caused by the elasticity of their midsole materials and by the fact that they elevate the foot off the ground. Some shoes offer greater stability than others, and some runners, namely overpronators, need it more than others. If you overpronate, you probably know it, but you can always have a shoe expert or podiatrist confirm it. Features to look for in a stability shoe are a medial post, a firm midsole, and a straight or semi-curved last. Severe overpronators and those with flat arches may need to supplement their motion control shoe with orthotics.

Socks

Like your cycling socks, your running socks should be light, low-cut, moisture-wicking, and protective in areas where blisters are most likely to occur. I like a thicker sock for running than I do for cycling, but some triathletes use the very same ones for both activities.

Shorts

Running short designs differ more than you might think. There are baggy shorts, split-seam, half-split, V-notch and full-seam shorts, short tights, shorts with a rear nutrition pocket, shorts with rugged fabric, shorts with and without drawstrings, and so forth. Don't just grab the first pair whose color you like. Different styles of running short fit and perform very differently. I've bought and received many a pair that I did not like.

Top

I'm appalled to see how many runners and triathletes still run in cotton T-shirts (even in marathons!) when so many breathable, moisture managing, and silky-feeling running tops are now available. You owe it to yourself to run in tops designed specifically for the activity of running. They will keep you cooler, drier, and more comfortable, and can even help you perform better. Whether you go for short sleeves, sleeveless tees, or tank tops is your call.

Sports Bra (Women)

I feel a bit weird, as a man, giving bra advice—even if it's sports bra advice—to women, but I have it on the authority of some very fine runners and triathletes with breasts that a good sports bra makes running far more comfortable. Go for support without constriction and a breathable, moisture-managing fabric. Note that, for racing, some (but only some) triathlon suits offer the support that larger-breasted women need for running.

Sports Watch

You'll want to time the majority of your swim, bike, and run workouts, but as pool clocks can cover the timing for swims, and as a bike computer can do the same for training rides, the sports watch is most essential for running. The qualities of a good sports watch for triathlon use are a large display, sweat and water resistance, multilap counter, easy-to-use stopwatch controls, and a good lighting system for when those long runs last beyond sundown.

Useful Run Stuff

Cold-Weather Apparel

I urge you to use only clothing designed for cold and wet running when running in the wet and cold. In cool autumn weather, regular running shorts or Lycra/spandex shorts and a long-sleeve base top should keep you comfortable. When the mercury drops to the low 40s or below, switch to tights and perhaps throw a thermal vest over your base top. In snow, wind, or bitter cold, switch to thicker tights and add running gloves, a hat or ear warmer, and perhaps a shell and storm pants. Or else wimp out and run indoors on a treadmill.

Racing Flats

Competitive triathletes use racing flats—super-light running shoes—in races and often in high-intensity run workouts as well. The same qualities that make for a good trainer make for a good racing flat, too, except that you can (and must) sacrifice some cushioning and/or stability in the latter due to the fact that you won't run in them as often or (usually) as far. Most triathletes choose not to use racing flats in Ironman-distance triathlons. If you're a serious overpronator, you may not be able to use racing flats at all.

Make sure to equip your racing flats with a speed lacing system such as that made by Gilly for faster bike-to-run transitions.

Hydration System

Any time you run for more than about an hour, you should carry water or a sports drink. In order to do this, you'll need to wear a hydration belt of some sort. Bottle bounce is the problem associated with the belts of lesser quality. The better belts avoid bottle bounce by angling the bottle pouch in back (which also makes removal and replacement easier) or by distributing holders for several small flasks (four to eight) around the belt. I advise against running with any kind of fluid bladder backpack because these can cause lower back problems.

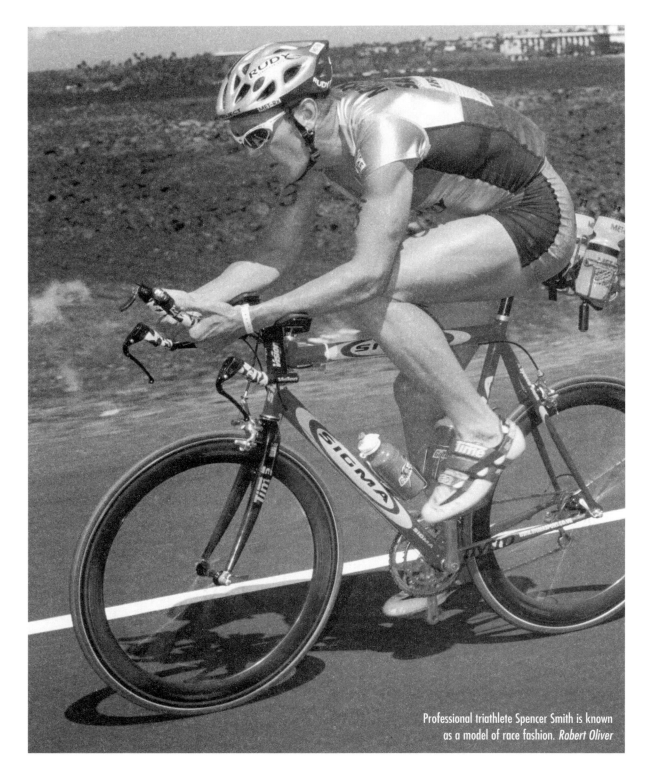

Professional triathlete Spencer Smith is known as a model of race fashion. *Robert Oliver*

Heart Rate Monitor

A heart rate monitor (as I'm sure you know) is a device that gives you a real-time reading of your pulse rate. Most monitors have two pieces: a transmitter located inside a strap that you wear around your upper torso, close to your heart, and a display watch that you wear around the wrist. Many triathletes use a heart rate monitor during most or all bike and run workouts as a way of gauging the intensity of their training. (There are some monitors you can swim in, but few swimmers and triathletes bother with them.)

The entry-level monitors offered by all the major manufacturers will do everything you really need a heart rate monitor to do. Fancier models allow you to do such things as download workout information onto your PC, which is a great feature, but not one that everyone wants to pay for. Things have gone wrong with a couple of the heart rate monitors I've owned, so I suggest looking into the warranty that comes with any model you might buy.

Looking Fast

In 1992, a nineteen-year-old Englishman named Spencer Smith burst onto the international triathlon scene by winning the ITU (International Triathlon Union) Junior World Championship, which he followed up with consecutive Senior World Championship titles in '93 and '94. Yet Smith's unique image made just as great an impact as his racing. His pugilist's mug and muscularity earned him the nickname "The Hulk," and the cockney-talking speedster seemed to put as much thought and planning into his racing attire as he put into actual race strategy. Disdaining the bikini look that reigned supreme at the time, he had his clothing sponsor, Speedo, design special square-cut skin suits in arresting colors that he wore with cowls and terminator sunglasses for a look that was truly intimidating.

"I don't want to look like everyone else out there," Smith told me once in an interview. "I want them to look like me! Looking different and looking the part has always been something that I like to do—to present myself in a different but professional way. A bit spicier, you know?"

Triathlon is an image sport. Functional innovation has led to new forms that give the sport a distinct style that many triathletes choose to cultivate for its own sake. This is a good thing. I think every triathlete should have Smith's attitude and should make an effort to look sharp when training and racing. Why not? Let's be frank: Triathlon training creates a very fine-looking body. One might as well dress it up in clothing and accessories (and from the fashion perspective, the bike definitely counts as an accessory) that *deserve* to adorn one's hard-earned physical form, rather than spoil the effect with careless shopping and indifferent dressing. To paraphrase haute couture maven Christian Dior, there's no such thing as an ugly triathlete, just a lazy triathlete.

Personal style, no matter how individual, is always based on general taste. So, the first step to take in cultivating your own triathlon look is to scrutinize other triathletes and single out the individuals whose look most appeals to you. Use these observations as fodder for reflection upon your personality and the manner of self-presentation that will be most consistent with it. And as with street clothing, go for colors that flatter your own coloring and cuts that accentuate your better attributes.

Triathlon fashion, for better or worse, is also every bit as much a brand thing as everyday fashion. Not all brands carry equal cachet. The coolest brands are frequently those that cater almost exclusively to triathletes. I won't name any of these brands for fear of excluding others, but it's not hard to discover them on your own. One way to really maximize the brand thing is to make yourself look "sponsored" by wearing a single brand's gear from head to toe.

Among the most common triathlon fashion faux pas are failing to match one's bike or running shoes with one's triathlon suit, wearing gym shorts and T-shirts for training runs, and, for men, failing to keep one's legs smoothly shaved at all times. Gotta shave those legs!

CHAPTER 3

Swim Training

Swimming is probably the reason there aren't more triathletes than there are. You might say it's triathlon's barrier discipline. Whereas inexperienced cyclists and runners generally need to overcome little more than a lack of confidence to gain momentum on two wheels and on their own two feet, inexperienced swimmers more often seem to face outright anxiety in the water. Indeed, most inexperienced swimmers (the adult ones, at least) would rather *remain* inexperienced swimmers. And this is why triathlon isn't about to overtake running in popularity anytime soon. However, it is interesting to note that the popularity of duathlon, which is triathlon minus the swim, pales in comparison to that of its close multisport cousin. So, swimming is clearly also a part of triathlon's attraction as well. People come to the sport in search of a diverse challenge, and swimming helps make it that.

Of course, just as many triathletes have a swimming background as have a cycling or a running background. But the majority of swimmers who become triathletes have a background in *pool* swimming, which is rather different from triathlon's long, open water swim format, and so pretty much every new triathlete faces a learning curve in relation to triathlon swimming, regardless of athletic background. This chapter makes no assumptions about your experience or proficiency as a swimmer, within or outside the context of triathlon. The one assumption I will make here is that you'd like to be a better triathlon swimmer, and there's only one path that leads in this general direction, however far along it you may be today.

The Nature of Swim Training

Bike and run training are far more similar to each other than standard swim training is to either one of them. Swim training tends to include more interval work and technique drills and significantly less long, slow distance. Also, the typical swim workout is more complex and varied, including several types of training, whereas cyclists and runners usually do just one type of training per workout session. Further, swimmers practice a different form of periodization than cyclists and runners do. Cyclists and runners generally practice something like linear periodization, wherein the various types of training are largely separated into distinct training phases. Swimmers, on the other hand, generally practice something more like nonlinear periodization, wherein the various training types are largely mixed together throughout the training cycle.

There are a few good justifications for the unique format of standard swim training. First of all, pool swimmers are mainly sprinters. The typical pool swim event lasts just a minute or two. And, indeed, standard swim training, with all its intervals, technique work, and variation, bears a closer resemblance to track and field sprint training than it bears to the regimen of a long-distance runner. Second, good technique is simply harder to come by in swimming, which not only necessitates the various technique drills employed, but also justifies the interval format, because shorter, faster swims promote good technique better than longer, slower swims. Third, the nature of swimming is such that more high-intensity training is feasible. Swimming does not elevate the heart rate or cause muscle tissue breakdown to the degree that cycling and especially running do, which allows swimmers to do longer and more frequent high-intensity workouts. And last, boredom is a bigger issue in swimming than in the less confined activities of cycling and running, which is another good justification for the variety and complexity that characterize the typical pool workout.

But again, triathlon swimming is rather different from pool racing. To start, the vast majority of triathlon swim legs take place in open water. More important, though, the average triathlon swim leg is much longer than the average pool race, and furthermore, triathletes must complete their swim with enough energy left in reserve to continue exercising for at least another hour or so, whereas the pool swimmer who's completed his or her race can be dragged out of the water and laid out on the deck, if necessary. Because of these differences, triathlon swim training is, or at least should be, distinct from standard pool training in certain ways. In particular, like competitive open water swimmers, triathletes need to do more endurance swimming (that is, long swims at a steady pace), some amount of which should take place in an actual open water environment. Also, triathletes can and should focus more specifically on the freestyle stroke than pool swimmers typically do.

Triathletes should base their swim training on the five-intensity system introduced in Chapter 1: recovery, endurance, threshold, max oxygen, and speed. Pool swimmers generally do not think about intensity levels that are associated with specific physiological states and training effects. More often, they simply think about the times they tend to shoot for when swimming intervals of various lengths. The main reason swimmers don't think about intensity in a physiological sense is that all of their races are mostly anaerobic. Because triathlon swims are almost entirely aerobic, triathletes have more reason to distinguish their above-threshold training from their below-threshold training. Also, using the five-intensity system helps triathletes give uniformity to their training across the three triathlon disciplines.

Beyond these points of distinction, however, triathletes should train more or less like pool swimmers (or, more specifically, like freestylers who specialize in the longer pool events)—which is to say, in the pool, doing drills and lots of intervals.

Group Versus Solo Swimming

Another factor that distinguishes swim training from bike and run training is that venues for swimming are almost infinitely more limited in number than venues for cycling and running. For this reason, competitive swimmers (and triathletes as swimmers) tend to congregate. And because they tend to find themselves in the same place at the same time doing more or less the same thing, they tend to form clubs and teams and perform structured group workouts led by designated coaches, much as youth swimmers do. In the United States, the majority of these clubs operate under the auspices of a single national organization, United States Masters Swimming,* which is dedicated to promoting fitness and competitive swimming among adults. In other countries, there are different kinds of clubs and teams, but no matter where you are, training within a formal group environment is far more common in swimming than in cycling or running.

*For more information about USMS, call (800) 550-SWIM or visit www.usms.org.

The advantages of training with a club or team are significant. First of all, you get a (presumably) knowledgeable coach who can design and lead sensible workouts and also scrutinize and help correct your technique. Additionally, you get the motivational boost that comes with structure, camaraderie, and the mild intraclub competition that's unavoidable in such an environment. And in most cases, you get all of this for very little money. Triathletes who train regularly with a Masters swim team or another formal group tend to train more consistently and harder than those who do not. For all of these reasons, I recommend that you do the majority of your training in this way, if it's at all convenient.

The average Masters workout lasts about 75 minutes and covers more than 3,000 yards (or meters), which is a fairly meaty training session.* So, if you're a comparatively weak swimmer, you'll want to spend some time developing a solid base of swim fitness before joining a group. If and when you feel you're ready to plunge into group workouts, take the following steps. First: Make sure you know basic workout structure, as well as how to read a pace clock, pool etiquette, and how to perform the most common drills (all of which topics I will cover in this chapter), as this practical knowledge will be expected of you. Second: Choose your group. In the United States, you can locate all the Masters swim programs in your area by perusing the "Places to Swim" section of the U.S. Masters Swimming Web site or by ordering a printed version of this directory for $9. You can locate any other local swim clubs or teams by contacting individual pool facilities. If there are several options, quiz your fellow triathletes to find out which among them will be the best match for you. Third: At your first workout, introduce yourself to the coach, briefly describe your swimming ability and goals, and ask him or her to point you to the appropriate lane (swimmers generally choose lanes based on their average 100-yard interval pace). Fourth: Swim the prescribed workout to the best of your ability, and make sure to solicit stroke advice from the coach in the event that none is volunteered. If, for any reason, you cannot complete the workout (as I could not complete my first Masters workout), just climb out of the pool and trust that you'll complete the next one, or the one after that (as I did).

---

* Lap pools come in four standard sizes—25 yards, 25 meters, 50 yards, and 50 meters. As the difference between a yard and a meter is small, most swimmers think of them as basically equal. For the sake of brevity, I'll refer to all distances in yards.

One thing to avoid with group workouts is allowing them to become your entire source of swim training. As a triathlete, you'll need to deviate from your team program in certain ways in order to stick to your own. For example, Masters groups never do long, steady-pace endurance swims, as you should do about once a week. In the sections on swim workouts and periodization of swim training below, I will present a set of guidelines for your triathlon swim training. Swim with your group as much as you like without departing from these guidelines, rather than follow the guidelines as much as you can without departing from your group. When you do attend group workouts, be prepared to do whatever the group does—modifications other than stopping early are disruptive and frowned upon. You can also customize the workout to some degree by choosing a slower or faster lane than usual.

Freestyle Technique

In virtually every elite-level freestyle swim race, the winner is he or she who takes the fewest total strokes. This is proof that swimming fast is not so much about moving your arms and legs fast, but about how far forward you move with each stroke taken. Distance per stroke is a function of power and hydrodynamics. The more directional force you're able to produce with your kick and, especially, your arm pull, the more distance you'll cover with each stroke. At the same time, the more streamlined your body is, the less water resistance it will encounter, and the more distance you'll cover with each stroke. Here are the elements of a powerful and streamlined freestyle technique:

Arm Cycle

The so-called *arm cycle* of the freestyle stroke comprises five segments: entry, catch, pull, release, and recovery. *Entry* is the segment of the arm cycle in which your hand enters the water. It should do so eight to 12 inches in front of your head and somewhere between the center of your head and the shoulder socket, from a lateral perspective. Your hand should be flat (fingers together) and angled at about 45 degrees to the surface of the water, with your palm turned slightly outward so that your thumb and index finger hit first. As this happens, extend your arm fully by reaching as far forward as you can, and at the same time rotate your forearm slightly so that your hand is now perfectly parallel to the surface of the pool, just beneath it. To increase your forward extension, roll your body to the side as you reach forward.

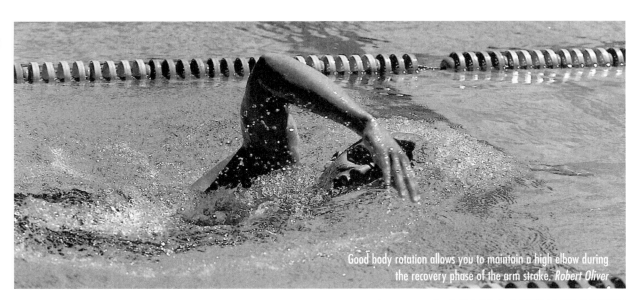

Good body rotation allows you to maintain a high elbow during the recovery phase of the arm stroke. *Robert Oliver*

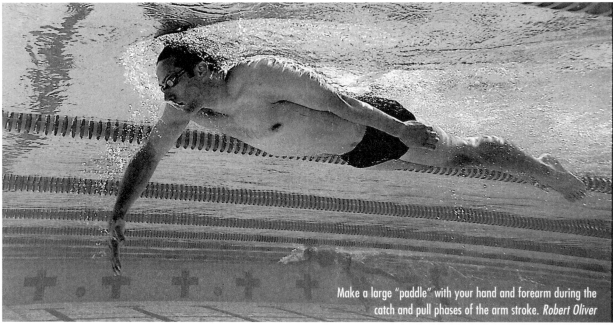

Make a large "paddle" with your hand and forearm during the catch and pull phases of the arm stroke. *Robert Oliver*

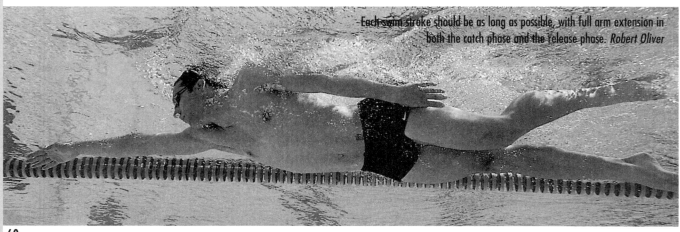

Each swim stroke should be as long as possible, with full arm extension in both the catch phase and the release phase. *Robert Oliver*

Entry leads into the *catch,* in which you rotate your shoulder downward and bend your elbow to 90 degrees in order to form a long paddle with your hand and forearm that will give you a much more powerful pull than the hand alone could provide. If you keep your arm straight for the pull, as many novice swimmers do, you'll be stuck with a small, hand-only paddle and will get a weaker pull. In the *pull* segment, keep your arm bent and, using your chest and back muscles, pull your paddle along the midline of your body toward your legs. Try to make this an accelerating movement, with the greatest application of force coming at the bottom of the pull. As your hand passes beneath your chest, straighten your arm once more to prepare for the release.

In the *release,* your hand exits the water at the point of full backward arm extension, next to your upper thigh. Releasing early, when the hand is next to the hipbone, is a common technique flaw. When releasing, rotate your palm toward your body so that your pinkie finger exits the water first. As this happens, turn your palm outward to prepare for the recovery. This movement minimizes shoulder strain in the release portion of the arm cycle. In the *recovery,* you carry your arm forward above the water to set up the next entry. It's important to do this in as relaxed a manner as possible, so as to avoid wasting energy on a portion of the stroke that produces no forward propulsion. Allow your hand and forearm to dangle and concentrate on carrying your elbow forward, until it comes even with your ear, at which point you will extend your arm once more and reach forward with your hand for the next entry.

So, that's one arm. In the freestyle stroke, the two arms are always at opposite points of the arm cycle. When one arm is catching, the other is releasing, and so forth.

Rotation

Rotation is the most important part of the stroke with respect to minimizing drag in the water. It also allows you to take longer and more powerful arm pulls. When the freestyle stroke is performed correctly, your entire body rotates from side to side, beginning with the shoulders and continuing along down to your feet in a fishlike fashion.

Rotation begins as you reach your hand forward at the end of the entry phase of the arm cycle. Think of the way you twist your torso away from your reaching hand in order to gain an extra inch or two of height when you try to grab something off a high shelf. You should rotate as much as 60 degrees to either side, which seems exaggerated to many beginners. The hips, legs, and feet follow the lead of your torso in rotating back to center during the pull phase of the arm cycle.

Body Position

When swimming freestyle, you want to float as high in the water as possible in order to minimize drag. Proper body position is that which optimizes float. The most common deviation from proper body position is sinking legs. You need to keep your feet within six inches of the water's surface and allow your chest to be the deepest part of your body. Maintaining this position is made easier when you position your head correctly, which involves looking just slightly forward (but mostly downward) when swimming and allowing the surface of the water to horizontally bisect your ears. Arching your neck back tends to cause the legs to drop and it also strains the neck and increases drag. Looking straight down can cause your legs to float too high.

Kick

In endurance swimming, the kick serves a minor role in propulsion (except during brief surges) and a greater role in maintaining stroke rhythm and proper body position. The form of kicking used in freestyle swimming is called the flutter kick. It involves making a small, up-and-down scissors motion in which the two legs are always moving in opposite directions, like the arms in running. A good kick is small in amplitude, very steady, and is initiated from the hips and buttocks rather than at the knee. Keep your toes pointed and flex the knee only slightly at the top of the kick.

Coordinating the kick with the arm cycle is a somewhat individual matter. The most popular kick in endurance swimming is the two-beat, in which the *left* leg kicks twice for each complete (entry-to-entry) cycle of the *right* arm. Some swimmers prefer a four-beat kick, while the six-beat kick is used only for sprinting and surging. Always try to increase the rate of your kick more than the size of it when sprinting or surging.

Breathing

It is important that you do not allow your stroke to interfere with your breathing, nor allow your breathing to interfere with your stroke. Exhalation occurs via forceful blowing through the mouth, underwater, as you stroke. When exhalation is complete, you inhale by turning your head just slightly at the top of your body rotation and sucking in all the air you can get during the brief moment when your face comes out of the water. This extra movement of the head should be as subtle as possible.

Less experienced swimmers tend to breathe always on the same side, every two or four strokes. Better swimmers practice bilateral breathing, constantly alternating the side on which they inhale, every three to five strokes. The main advantage of being able to breathe on both sides is that it promotes symmetrical swim mechanics. But there are additional advantages in open water, where the ability to breathe on either side allows you to sight better and avoid swallowing water in choppy conditions. You should definitely make it a point to learn bilateral breathing by practicing it for a few lengths at a time until it becomes second nature.

Improving Technique

There are four main ways of improving freestyle swim technique. The first of these is *emulation*. Nobody performs proper freestyle technique naturally, by instinct—its present form represents the culmination of a long evolutionary process in which many small refinements have been contributed by athletes and coaches. Emulation is facilitated by reading descriptions of freestyle technique, as you've just done, and by analyzing the technique of advanced swimmers in photographs, on video, and in person. A second means of improving technique, which follows naturally from emulation, is *kinesthetic awareness.* This involves simply concentrating on technique as you swim, rather than allowing your mind to wander. You have the choice of concentrating on just one portion of the stroke for some time, allowing your attention to roam from one portion of the stroke to another, or concentrating on how the whole thing comes together. I recommend doing all three, although beginners may need to emphasize the first of these options.

A third means of improving your freestyle technique is to have your stroke analyzed. Indeed, after plain old time in the water, *stroke analysis* is probably the single most indispensable tool for becoming a better swimmer. You cannot possibly self-diagnose and self-correct every single flaw in your stroke. Even Olympians rely on others for this. As I said above, Masters swim coaches are a great resource for stroke analysis. They can provide it both within the context of group workouts or one-on-one (sometimes for an additional fee, sometimes not—it depends on the coach). Another good way to receive stroke analysis is by attending a weekend swim or triathlon camp, some of which even offer videotape stroke analysis. You can also do your own videotaping and send the tape to an expert coach for analysis by mail.

And then there are the *technique drills,* most of which involve neutralizing one part of the stroke or another so that the swimmer can concentrate on another part. Here are descriptions of the most effective technique drills:

Catch-up Drill

This drill modifies the normal freestyle stroke such that you move only one arm at a time. Begin with both arms outstretched in front of you. Perform a complete arm cycle with either arm, while kicking normally (preferably wearing fins—see below—to keep your speed up). When the cycling arm rejoins the other, hold it there while performing a complete cycle with the second arm. This drill improves technique in all phases of the arm cycle.

Count Stroke Drill

Simply count the number of strokes you take while swimming one complete length of the pool with normal freestyle technique, and then try to lower the number of strokes taken in each of two or three subsequent lengths. You will achieve this by taking longer, more powerful pulls, rotating more, and allowing yourself to glide a little bit. Don't be afraid to exaggerate these elements in order to decrease the stroke count. This drill helps to improve overall stroke efficiency.

Fingertip Drag Drill and Thumb Scrape Drill

Swim a normal freestyle stroke, except consciously drag your fingertips across the surface of the water during the recovery phase. This modification helps you relax and use as little energy as possible during the recovery phase of the arm cycle. The Fingertip Drag Drill can be performed in conjunction with the Thumb Scrape Drill, in which you purposely scrape your thumb against your thigh during the release phase of the arm cycle. This modification promotes complete arm extension and proper hand position in the release.

Fist Drill

Swim with your fists clenched. This drill teaches you to rotate your shoulder and bend your elbow in the catch portion of the arm cycle in order to create a powerful paddle for the pull. If you do this correctly, you will swim with only slightly less power than you do with open hands.

Kick on Side Drill

Swim half a length on either side with your bottom arm extended in front of you and your top arm resting on your surface side. Propel yourself by kicking only. After completing half a length, rotate to the other side and complete the length. This drill allows you to focus on kick technique and promotes better rotation. I recommend wearing fins while doing it.

Other Skills

In addition to freestyle technique, there is a grab bag of other skills you'll need to develop in your swim training. These include reading the pace clock, alternative strokes, flip turns, pool etiquette, using swim aids, and open water swimming.

Reading the Pace Clock

Most lap pools have one or more large pace clocks set up in highly visible places. When you swim alone, you can choose whether or not you wish to use the pace clock to time intervals and recoveries. In group workouts, you will have to do so. The clock has a minute hand and a second hand. Interval sets are usually prescribed in the following manner: "Do 10 x 50 freestyle on the one-minute." This means that you will perform 10 individual 50-yard swims, and that you will begin each of the last nine when the second hand reaches the spot it was at when you began the first (which will most often be the top of the clock, marked "60"). So, the portion of each minute that is accounted for by rest depends on how quickly you complete each 50-yard swim. If, for example, you complete your first 50-yard swim in 50 seconds, you will rest 10 seconds before beginning your second swim.

Alternative Strokes

Even as a triathlete, you should learn how to do a rudimentary backstroke and breaststroke. Many workouts call for the use of alternative strokes as a means of active recovery between sets, or between intervals within a set, and with good justification. Both strokes (sometimes referred to as off-strokes) use the muscles differently than freestyle does, so they give your freestyle muscles a good rest even as you remain active, thereby flushing lactic acid from your back and shoulders while lowering your heart rate gradually. Because you're not shooting for speed in either of these strokes, it's okay to learn them casually by imitating fellow swimmers who do them well. As for the butterfly stroke —well, there's just no such thing as a casual butterfly.

Flip Turns

Sooner or later, you need to learn how to perform a flip turn. Using flip turns allows you to swim more steadily than using open turns, in which you grab the wall with one hand or both hands, pull your feet to it, and then push off with your head above the water. Using flip turns also allows you to swim faster splits and therefore train with faster swimmers, who can pull you along to further improvement.

The flip turn has three phases: the approach, the flip, and the push-off. The key to the approach is judging when to initiate the turn. This just takes practice. The idea is to determine which stroke is to be your last before you flip. Also, make sure to inhale right before this final stroke so that you can exhale during the flip, which will prevent your getting water up the nose. Stop stroking with one arm extended in front of you (post-entry) and the other extended down along your side (pre-release). In preparation for the flip, pull your forward arm down along your other side.

Next, do a forward roll underwater, while still moving forward. Your butt should break the surface of the water, followed by your lower legs. Try to flip "through" your arms, like immobile wickets, and "leave" them extended away from the wall, in position for a streamlined push-off. As you complete your somersault, you should find yourself facing the surface of the water. When your feet make contact with the wall, allow your knees to bend deeply to absorb impact and prepare you for a powerful push-off.

Push away from the wall hard with both legs. As you glide forward and rise toward the surface, rotate back toward your stomach. When your hands break the surface, begin stroking.

Pool Etiquette

The basic rules for solo lap swimming are as follow. One: Always choose an empty lane if one's available. Two: If no empty lanes are available, choose a lane that is occupied by a swimmer who appears to be swimming at a pace close to yours. Three: Don't interrupt this swimmer to announce your decision to enter the lane. Just climb in on the right side of the lane and allow the swimmer to notice you. If the person stops, ask whether he or she would prefer to split the lane or circle. If the swimmer begins circling or chooses one side automatically, follow suit. Four: When you are joined in a lane by another swimmer, acknowledge his or her presence by choosing one side of the lane or by starting to circle it counterclockwise, keeping to the right. Five: Whenever three swimmers share a lane, circling is mandatory. Six: When passing another swimmer, tap his or her left foot with your right hand and go around on the left. If this person knows pool etiquette, he or she will take the tap as a signal to slow for a moment and allow you to pass. Seven: If you get tapped on the foot, slow down and allow the other swimmer to pass.

Here are the basic rules of group workouts. One: Circle swim in counterclockwise fashion, keeping to the right. Two: Tap to pass. Three: If you pass or get stuck behind another swimmer during an interval, ask this person whether you can leave before him or her on the next interval. Four: If you get passed, allow this person to take your spot for the next interval. Five: Don't draft off another swimmer throughout a workout. Six: Always leave on your designated interval. Don't leave early to draft or leave late for extra rest. Seven: Choose the right lane! If you're finishing your intervals too quickly, you're cheating yourself by getting too much rest between intervals. If you're finishing your intervals too slowly, you're probably cheating others by bottlenecking your lane.

Using Swim Aids

Four devices, categorized as swim aids, are commonly used in swim training: fins, paddles, kickboards, and pull buoys. Swimmers and triathletes use swim fins to develop a more powerful kick and to develop the muscles and joints used in the kicking motion, as well as to maintain speed while performing technique drills such as the Catch-up Drill. Although not an essential item, fins will improve your swimming, if used properly (and not excessively), so I recommend them. Wear fins for one or two weekly sets of power intervals during the first half of the base phase, which is the best time to work on strength and power, and then limit their use to one or two drill sets a week for the remainder of the training cycle. When you buy a pair, make sure to get fins that are designed specifically for swim training rather than traditional scuba fins, which are much longer and encourage big, slow kicks that will wreak havoc upon your freestyle form.

Swim paddles are to the hands as swim fins are to the feet. They extend the surface area of the hand and thereby increase the amount of water resistance you must overcome with each stroke, which promotes the development of stronger muscles and joints. Paddles are best avoided by less advanced swimmers, however, as they can quickly lead to tendinitis of the shoulder if used with flawed technique. If you've never used them before, start with a smaller pair (they come in sizes) and use them for just a few intervals, and build from there. As with the other power swim aid, swim fins, you should do the greatest amount of swimming with paddles during the first half of the base phase and limit their use to within one or two drill sets a week thereafter.

The most commonly used swim aid, kickboards are simple flotation devices that allow you to just kick without sinking. Like fins, kickboards are used to improve kick power, but they are not as effective as fins for this purpose and they also eliminate the body rotation that is a fundamental component of good freestyle technique. Whereas fins are for all swimmers and paddles are mostly for experienced swimmers, kickboards are primarily a beginner's aid. Even beginners should avoid making a crutch of them, however.

Finally, the pull buoy is to the legs as the kickboard is to the arms. It's a flotation device that keeps your legs afloat without kicking so you can concentrate on your pull technique. I do not recommend its use because it, too, eliminates body rotation.

Open Water Swimming

Open water swimming is essential practice for triathletes and often a fun break from the monotony of the pool. However, lakes and oceans are less controlled environments than pools and present some challenges for which you need to be prepared.

Choose your open water venues carefully. Swim where people swim. Other places can have dangerous rip tides or contaminants that you don't know about. For that matter, even swimming beaches can be plagued periodically by conditions (storms or sewage runoff for instance) that make swimming dangerous or impossible, so always check into the present and imminent conditions of your chosen venue before plunging in.

The ideal open water venue is placid, free of obstructions like algae and motorized traffic, not too cold, and lifeguard-protected. Buoys at marked distances are a nice bonus. Always know where and how far you will swim before starting, and make sure you and your swimming partners are on the same page. Try to avoid swimming more than a half mile or so from shore, and never swim solo unless very close to shore or in popular areas where other swimmers are always nearby.

When the water is cooler than about 65 degrees, you may want to wear a wetsuit. Avoid swimming in water that is colder than 55 degrees or so, even with a wetsuit. If you wear a full wetsuit in water that is warmer than 68 degrees, not only are you a wimp, but in all likelihood you'll also overheat. If you plan to compete in a wetsuit, you need to practice swimming in it and taking it off, especially as a beginner.

Sighting is an important skill in open water swimming and one you'll definitely want to practice, because if you can't sight, you can't swim in a straight line. It's very simple in concept. The idea is to look forward periodically and find the buoy or landmark you're swimming toward to determine whether you are, in fact, swimming toward it. The key to sighting well is sighting often. Nobody swims in a straight line blind. You should check your bearing every few strokes. When sighting, look forward at the *bottom* of your rotation (just enough to get your goggles above water), spot your target, and then twist your head to the side and breathe as you reach maximum body rotation to that same side. Triathletes should practice doing this in the pool as well as in open water.

You'll also want to take advantage of your open water workouts to practice entering and exiting, especially if you compete in the ocean, with surf. Practice charging into the water, diving forward, and swimming very hard for 50 yards before settling into race pace. In crowded swim starts, it pays to get out ahead if you're fit enough to do so. If there's surf, practice diving under incoming waves and pushing off the sandy bottom behind them. Then turn around and practice exiting. Swim right up until your hand touches sand before standing. Then run onto the beach and begin to remove your wetsuit, if you're wearing one. Again, if there's surf, practice timing the waves so you can body surf to shore. I've seen triathletes gain 50 yards this way in races.

Swim Workouts

For triathletes, there are two basic types of swim workout: steady-pace endurance swims and interval workouts. The typical swim workout contains a warm-up, a set of drill intervals, a main interval set, and a cool-down. The drill set is usually forgone in endurance swims, and nobody does them in open water. Some group swim interval workouts may include a separate sprint set before or after the main set, and may also include a second set of drills preceding the cool-down. However, in the workouts I prescribe, for the sake of simplicity, these options are not included.

Interval workouts are classified by three types. Short interval workouts contain intervals ranging between 25 and 100 yards in their main set. Long interval workouts contain intervals ranging between 100 and 600 yards in their main set. Mixed interval workouts contain—you guessed it—a mix of short and long intervals in their main set. In accordance with the nonlinear periodization model that works best for swim training, you should try to perform some amount of short intervals, long intervals, and steady-pace endurance swimming each week throughout the training cycle. If you swim only twice a week, you can approximate this ideal by performing one endurance swim per week and cycling through short, long, and mixed interval workouts for your second weekly swim. If you swim three times a week, do an endurance swim and any combination of the three interval workout types. If you swim more than three times, do one endurance swim, at least one short interval workout, and at least one long interval workout. Following are guidelines for each of the components of swim workouts:

Warm-up and Cool-down

The warm-up and cool-down generally should consist of easy freestyle swimming at recovery or endurance pace (see the section on intensity below). The warm-up warms, lubricates, and loosens the muscles, which prepares them for the hard work to follow, while the cool-down flushes metabolic wastes from the muscles and prepares them for a speedy recovery. In other words, the warm-up and cool-down fulfill very important functions and should never be skipped. Your warm-up should last at least 10 minutes and your cool-down at least 5.

Drill Set

In the drill portion of a swim workout, you should perform two to four technique and/or power drills in interval structure. The total distance covered in this portion of the workout should be 300 to 500 yards. Here are some sample drill sets:

DRILL SET #1

8 x 25 Kick on Side Drill w/ 0:10 rest
4 x 50 Count Stroke Drill w/ 0:05 rest

DRILL SET #2

4 x (25 Fist Drill, 25 Catch-up Drill) w/ 0:15 rest
4 x 50 pull w/ paddles w/ 0:05 rest

You should strive for variety in your drill sets, but give primary emphasis to the specific drills that address your particular stroke flaws. For example, if you have a tendency to use a straight-arm pull, repeat the Fist Drill often. Drill time is a good time to strap on fins so you can maintain speed and work on kick power while you address your stroke issues.

Main Set

There's no limit to the variety of main sets you can construct using the variables at your disposal. While it's possible to found an effective triathlon swim program on just a handful of individual workouts, many coaches and athletes try to test their creativity in main set construction,[*]

* For example, triathlon coach Roch Frey keeps a database of nearly 400 individual workouts that he prescribes to clients and administers in Masters swim workouts.

for two reasons. First, in swimming, varying the nature of the demands you place on your body is a key means of stimulating progressive gains in fitness. And second, more variation means less boredom. Here's a look at the major variables that are manipulated in main set construction:

Intensity

Training the right amount at the right intensity levels is essential to achieving the desired training effects from these workouts. Your training should involve five basic swim paces, each of which correlates with one of the five intensity levels (recovery, endurance, threshold, max oxygen, and speed) discussed in Chapter 1. Recovery pace is easy and comfortable, although still fast enough to qualify as exercise, and is appropriate for warm-ups, cool-downs, and active recoveries. Endurance pace is slightly faster—hard enough to leave you moderately fatigued at the end of your long endurance swims, which will last 40 minutes to two hours, depending on your fitness level and goals. Threshold pace is the swimming intensity just above which your muscles begin to rapidly accumulate lactic acid. Max oxygen pace is the swimming pace at which your body saturates its capacity to consume oxygen. Speed pace does not correlate to any specific physiological threshold, but is simply 5 to 10 percent faster than max oxygen pace.

Determining your present training pace levels is not difficult. The key is simply to perform appropriately structured main sets, because when you do so, it's hard *not* to swim at the right intensity. Generally, intervals of 25 to 50 yards in length are most appropriate for speed pace, intervals of 100 to 200 yards are most appropriate for max oxygen pace, and intervals of 200 to 400 yards (or even 600 yards, for highly fit triathletes) are most appropriate for threshold pace. Your speed pace is the fastest pace you can maintain through a full set of 25- or 50-yard intervals without slowing down in the last one or two. Your max oxygen pace is the fastest pace you can maintain through a full set of 100- to 200-yard intervals without slowing down in the final intervals. And your threshold pace is the fastest pace you can maintain through a full set of 200- to 400-yard intervals without slowing down in the last interval or developing substantial lactic acid burn in your shoulders. When you wish to emphasize endurance intensity, don't do intervals at all, but instead perform a steady-pace endurance workout. Now, these guidelines only work if you perform the right number of intervals with respect to your fitness level and the purpose of the workout and rest neither too short nor too long between repetitions. I'll address these factors momentarily.

Suggested Swim Training Paces

Recovery	Endurance	Threshold	Max O$_2$	Speed
(per 100)	(per 100)	(per 100)	(per 100)	(per 50)
1:16	1:12	1:03	1:00	0:28
1:22	1:18	1:08	1:05	0:31
1:28	1:24	1:13	1:10	0:33
1:34	1:30	1:19	1:15	0:36
1:40	1:36	1:25	1:20	0:38
1:46	1:42	1:30	1:25	0:40
1:52	1:48	1:35	1:30	0:43
1:58	1:54	1:41	1:35	0:46
2:04	2:00	1:46	1:40	0:48
2:10	2:06	1:51	1:45	0:50
2:16	2:12	1:56	1:50	0:53
2:22	2:18	2:01	1:55	0:56
2:28	2:24	2:28	2:00	0:58

Table 3.1

Table 3.1 is designed to help you find the appropriate pace for each intensity level. If you're able to determine your pace per 100 yards (or per 50 yards, in the case of speed intensity) for any one of the five training intensities, you can use this table to obtain a suggested pace for each of the other four. These suggested pace targets may not be perfect, but they should be very close. Individual swimmers who share the same max oxygen pace should train at roughly the same pace at all five intensity levels, because the same two variables that determine one's max oxygen pace—VO$_2$ max and economy—also determine one's pace at the other four intensity levels. You can refine these estimates simply by performing appropriately structured workouts. If any given pace is slightly too easy or too hard, tweak it accordingly. And even if these suggested pace targets are perfect for you today, they will change—that is, improve—throughout the training cycle as your swim fitness increases, so you should always be prepared to tweak.

Length and Number of Intervals

The lengths of the intervals you swim in any given main set should depend mostly on the intensity level or levels you wish to emphasize. As I suggested above, intervals of 25 to 50 yards in length are most appropriate for speed pace, intervals of 100 to 200 yards are most appropriate for max oxygen pace, and intervals of 200 to 400 yards (or even 600 yards, for highly fit triathletes) are most appropriate for threshold pace, while steady, unbroken swims of 1,000 to 5,000 yards are the best way to train at endurance intensity. The number of intervals you perform should vary inversely in proportion to the length of the intervals (assuming a main set containing intervals of uniform length). For example, a main set comprised of 50s should contain at least eight and as many as 20 intervals, whereas a main set comprised of 400s should contain no more than 5 or 6 intervals. Naturally, your present fitness level and the length of your peak race should be the primary determinants of the precise number of intervals you choose to swim within the appropriate range. See Table 3.2 for suggested main set lengths for triathletes of various categories.

Rest

There are two kinds of rest in swim workouts: *passive recovery,* which entails holding on to the wall and gathering yourself between intervals, and *active recovery,* in which you swim easily, often using alternative strokes or just kicking, between hard efforts. Active recovery is most appropriate between subsets within a main set, when you wish to clear lactic acid out of the muscles in preparation for another hard subset. For example, consider the following threshold-pace main set: 3 x (4 x 100). In such a main set, you might take short (say, 20-second) passive recoveries after each 100, except every fourth, after which you might swim another 100 at recovery pace.

Passive recoveries can last as little as five seconds or as long as three minutes, depending on what you've just done and what you're doing next. Because longer rests allow you to swim harder afterward, and because shorter rests help your body learn to need less rest, you should use both. Typical rest durations are 20 to 40 seconds after speed intervals, 90 seconds to two minutes after max oxygen intervals, and 30 to 90 seconds after threshold intervals. The main functions of rest are to lower the heart rate to endurance-pace level and to flush accumulated lactic acid from the working muscles. Lactic acid concentrations are greatest after longer max oxygen intervals and after several speed intervals with short rests. This is why longer rests are typical after individual max oxygen intervals and why it is common and advisable to break speed sets into subsets that permit a fuller recovery after a few speed intervals.

Remember, in group workouts, your rest intervals will vary depending on how fast you swim each interval, as the prescribed interval time for each lane accounts for swimming and rest (otherwise it would be impossible to keep all swimmers in any single lane in sync).

Sample Main Sets

For each of these workouts, triathletes who are less fit and/or training for shorter events should perform closer to the minimum number and length of recommended intervals, while triathletes who are more fit and/or training for longer events should perform closer to the maximum number and length.

THRESHOLD MAIN SETS

Option 1: 4–12 x 200 w/ 0:30 rest
Option 2: 2–6 x 400 w/ 0:45 rest

MAX OXYGEN MAIN SETS

Option 1: 4–10 x 200 w/ 1:00 rest
Option 2: 3–6 x 300 w/ 2:00 rest

SPEED MAIN SETS

Option 1: 2–4 x (4 x 50 w/ 0:20 rest) w/ 100 swim recovery
Option 2: 2–4 x (100, 50, 25, 25 w/ 0:30 rest)

MIXED SETS

Option 1: (500), 400, 300, 200, 100 w/ 0:30 rest
(The parentheses indicate that the 500 is optional. Pace should increase as distance decreases.)
Option 2: 8–12 x 25 w/ 0:20 rest + 2–6 x 100 w/ 0:10 rest
(The 25s should be sprints. Swim the 100s at max oxygen pace.)

ENDURANCE SWIM

1,000–5,000
(This is just a long, steady swim at a moderate pace, or a variable pace that never becomes too intense.)

Swim Training Guidelines for Triathletes

Peak Race Type	Main Set (yards)	Total Swim (yards)	Weekly Swims
First Triathlon	400–800	800–1,500	2–3
Sprint	750–1,200	1,500–2,500	3
Middle	1,000–2,000	2,000-4,000	3–4
Long-Distance	1,500–3,000	3,000–6,000	4–5

Table 3.2

Periodization of Swim Training

Here's how I recommend approaching swim training in each of the three phases of the training cycle. I will discuss how to mix together swim, bike, and run training in each of the phases in Chapter 6.

Base Phase

Your swim training in the base phase should emphasize basic endurance, technique, and power. Begin the phase with a lower volume of swimming and increase it gradually and steadily throughout the phase in the step-loading manner (i.e., increase volume for two or three weeks, reduce volume for one week). By no later than the middle of this phase, start doing a weekly long endurance swim. Increase the duration of this workout by 5 to 10 percent every week or two weeks.

To increase the power of your swim stroke, in at least the first few weeks of the phase do as much as 15 percent of your total yardage using fins and 15 percent with paddles (never use both together) in the context of short intervals or drill sets. Make the drill set portion of your interval workouts fairly lengthy in the first few weeks of the base phase, focusing on the technique drills that are most beneficial for you. In the latter half of the phase, you may reduce the volume of swimming accounted for by technique and power drills and increase the volume accounted for by regular intervals. Do a mixture of threshold-pace, max-oxygen-pace, and speed-pace intervals.

Build Phase

In the build phase, it's time to do your hardest swimming with one objective in mind: getting faster. The base phase has prepared you for the challenging workouts you'll do here; the challenging workouts you do here will prepare you to do your most race-specific workouts in the coming peak phase.

Hold your overall swim training volume more or less constant (but continue to use step cycles) throughout the build phase while pushing yourself to the limit in at least one interval set each week. Hold steady the duration of your weekly long endurance swim as well. If you swim four to five times per week, push the pace in two of these workouts. Put the greatest emphasis on max-oxygen-pace intervals, but don't neglect the threshold and speed intensity levels. Pay attention to your splits and try to improve them gradually throughout the phase.

Peak Phase

Your swim training becomes most race-specific in this phase. Put the greatest emphasis on threshold-pace intervals, except during race weeks, when you should emphasize speed-pace intervals for sharpness. If you are training for a longer peak triathlon, begin to gradually increase the duration of your weekly endurance swim once again, until it's at least 25 percent longer than the swim leg of your peak triathlon (but no more than three miles). Reduce the frequency of your long endurance swims to once every other week; on the alternate weeks, do a shorter, race-pace swim. In the final two to four weeks before your most important race, you should eliminate endurance swims, reduce total volume, and maintain peak fitness with a small amount of high-intensity swimming.

Fast Company

Birds of a feather, as they say, flock together. In other words, individuals with common interests have a way of finding each other and sharing their pursuit of these interests. This is a good thing, because shared pursuit of common interests frequently yields a level of progress for each involved individual that could not have been achieved otherwise. Literary salons are a good example of this phenomenon. It's amazing to see how many of history's great writers nourished their growth toward creative heights by gathering with other talented writers once a week or so and reading their work, hearing the work of others, and discussing it and other relevant topics until the wee hours.

Individual sports like triathlon are no different than the arts in this regard. Triathletes who train in groups consistently achieve greater improvement than those who go it alone day in and day out. The reason is that it's easier to train harder in a group, where there's always someone pushing you from behind and pulling you from ahead. The difference between the effort you give alone and the effort you give in a group may be very small, but it's crucial, because barriers come down in those brief moments in workouts when you go *just a bit* further or faster.

Training in groups is also fun. It promotes greater overall enjoyment of the sport, which is both intrinsically good and also benefits bottom-line performance. It helps to develop and strengthen relationships with fellow triathletes, making the sport more than just a hobby but a lifestyle. For these reasons, I recommend that you make every reasonable effort to train in a social environment. Following are a few common ways of doing so:

Group Swim Workouts. As I mentioned above, many pool facilities host Masters swim programs and other group swim programs that gather for several formal workout sessions every week.

Triathlon/Cycling Clubs. In many areas there are formal triathlon and cycling clubs that offer dues-paying members group workout opportunities, coaching, and other benefits.

Group Rides/Runs. Less formal than clubs are the various group runs and rides that tend to begin at a regular place and time each week; they are free and welcome all comers.

Health Clubs. Health clubs are natural places to train socially and meet others who share your passion for endurance sports. Indoor group cycling classes are an especially fruitful forum in this regard.

Coach-Led Training Groups. Many areas are fortunate to have top-notch endurance coaches who lead regular group workouts (particularly in running) for a small fee. They offer all the advantages of a Masters swim program.

CHAPTER 4

Bike
Training

Cycling may be one of three triathlon disciplines, but it's really half the sport when considered from the perspective of time. Cycling accounts for about 50 percent of one's finishing time in a typical triathlon, and it should account for a similar percentage of one's training time. Cycling is therefore the costliest of the three disciplines to be weak in and the most favorable to have as a strong suit. There is more room for improvement in cycling than in swimming or running and greater opportunity to gain time on your age group rivals. The goal of this chapter is to help you make cycling a strong suit—or, at least, not a weakness.

The Nature of Bike Training

Conventional wisdom holds that the key to becoming a better cyclist is "time in the saddle." Of course, putting in time is vital to becoming a better swimmer and runner, too, but with cycling it's a little different. In swimming, technique is so important that half an hour spent refining technique is worth several hours of swimming for fitness with poor technique. In cycling, however, pure lung power and leg power can overcome less than perfect technique, and lungs and legs come with miles. In running, because the activity is so high-impact, the point of diminishing returns in terms of training volume is more quickly reached, so it's important to make every mile count. (Elite swimmers and cyclists train

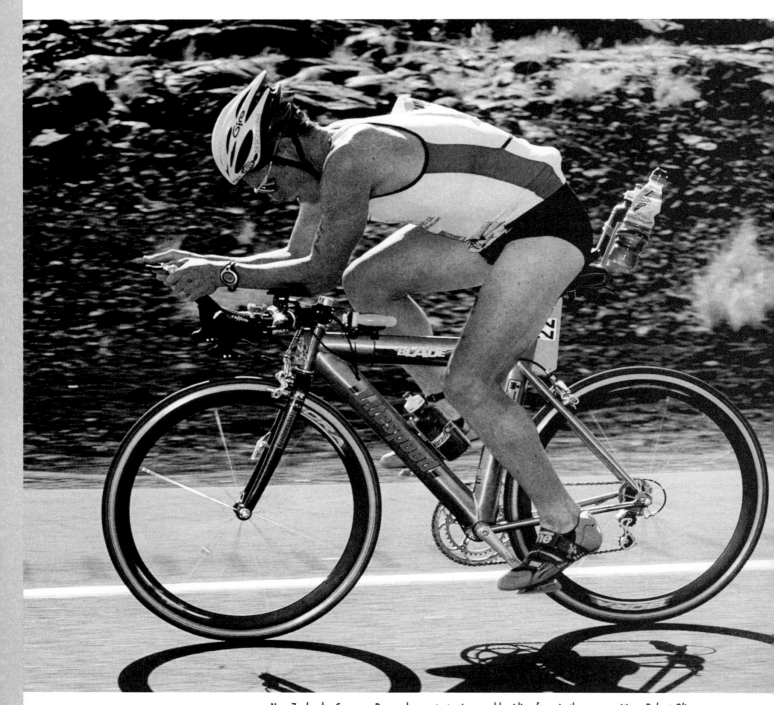

New Zealander Cameron Brown demonstrates impeccable riding form in the aero position. *Robert Oliver*

upward of six hours a day, whereas elite distance runners train "only" about 90 minutes a day.) In cycling, on the other hand, as long as you take proper precautions, you can ride almost endlessly without getting injured, and the cyclist who rides endlessly with no particular plan will always wind up being stronger than the cyclist who logs modest mileage with scientific precision.

This is not to say that exactly *how* one trains on the bike is unimportant, or that working on skills and technique is not also an excellent means of improving cycling performance, especially for those of us whose training time is limited. Making the best use of one's time in the saddle, however much it is, entails doing carefully selected workouts in the proper sequence while actively cultivating all the skills that are relevant to performance. But there is no substitute for sheer volume in bike training.

A second feature that makes bike training distinct from other forms of endurance training is the bike itself. A major factor in cycling performance is the ability to get the most out of a fairly complex machine. Developing as a cyclist is about "becoming one" with your bike, and the road. If you're at all experienced as a cyclist, you know just what I mean. You need to know how to position yourself on the bike, when to shift gears, how to keep the bike in race-ready condition, and so forth. The cooperation between human and machine, and the particular nature of this cooperation, also makes the nature of cycling fitness somewhat different from swim and run fitness. Speed on the bike is a function of pedaling cadence and of distance traveled per pedal stroke, which is a function of gear selection. The higher the gear you can push at a relatively high cadence for a long time, the faster you can go. Pushing higher gears is made possible by sheer muscular strength in the legs. Cycling fitness therefore has a greater strength component than either running or swimming. Cyclists and triathletes get the leg strength they need from climbing hills and training in high gears, and sometimes also from supplemental resistance training.

There are two major disciplines within the sport of road cycling: road racing and time trialing. Road racing entails pack riding, in which drafting is a major factor and the race is strictly against other riders rather than against the clock. Triathlon cycling takes place in a time trial format (except in World Cup races, in which only a fraction of 1 percent of triathletes ever participate), where drafting is illegal and the race is against the clock. For this reason, triathletes need to focus more on aerodynamic efficiency and on cultivating the ability to maintain a very steady pace at high intensity. At the same time, unlike even those pure cyclists who specialize in time trialing, triathletes must train themselves to conserve energy at high intensity, so as to be able to run between three and 26.2 miles at maximum effort as soon as they dismount from their bikes.

Fit and Riding Position

This process of becoming one with your bike begins with bike fit and riding position. Now, bike fit and riding position are the kinds of things mechanical geniuses engage in heated arguments about and Tour de France cyclists tinker with throughout their careers. They're part science, part art, and very complex. However, while you could tear your hair out trying to discover the *perfect* riding position, finding a perfectly good one is not nearly so challenging.

There are two ways to do it: with professional help, or on your own. I recommend both. A true bike-fitting expert can suggest refinements in your riding position that you would never think of, especially if you're a beginner, but even if you're a Cat II* stud. Just make sure you have it done by someone who understands triathlon cycling. But you can't run to an expert every time you need to make an adjustment, so you also should have the confidence to fit yourself without assistance, whether or not you ever pursue the first option (which isn't cheap, by the way—expect to pay at least $100, unless you're buying a bike, in which case it's free). This ability will help you move from bike to bike when necessary or modify your position on a given bike to suit circumstances. For example, many triathletes and cyclists tweak their riding position a few times during the course of a training cycle as their muscles develop. Triathletes, in particular, tend to move from a more relaxed aero position at the start of the season to a more extreme one by season's end. This is when a little bike-fitting knowledge comes in handy.

Basic fitting is not terribly difficult. First of all, always set up your bike for your *primary* riding position. If you have an aerobar, either on a triathlon bike or a road bike, set up the bike to optimize the aero position. If you're riding a road bike without a clip-on aerobar, set it up to optimize the hands-on-brake-hoods position. Either way, begin by setting the saddle height. If you use an aerobar, adjust it such that, when you're wearing cycling shoes, the *arch* of your shoe just barely touches the pedal when your knee is fully extended and the pedal is positioned at the bottom of the rotation. For a road bike without aerobar, set the

* Category II. Road cyclists compete in four categories. Category IV (or "Cat IV") cyclists are average competitors; Cat I riders are world-class.

saddle height such that the *heel* of your shoe touches the pedal (this will place the saddle just a few millimeters higher to account for the slightly slacker hip angle maintained in the road position). Make sure not to tilt your hips when performing this test.

Here's where aero fitting and road bike fitting diverge. Let's first focus on the aero position. The next step is to set your seat setback (or "fore-aft position," as some call it). To do this, clip into a pedal and rotate it to the three o'clock position. For this to work, you should have your shoe cleats already positioned exactly where you want them. Drop a plumb line (a string with a washer tied to one end works nicely) from the head of your fibula (the bony protrusion on the outside of the knee). If the string is in line with the pedal axle, your saddle is in the neutral position. Put the saddle in this position for now.

In the standard aero position, your torso will be almost perfectly parallel to the ground and your shoulders will be almost directly above (just slightly behind) your elbows. Adjust the aerobar (integrated or clip-on) to achieve this position. This will involve playing with both the height and the reach of the aerobar, at least, and may require further tweaking of the saddle setback, either slightly forward or slightly backward from the neutral position. If, after playing with all three of these settings, your position still isn't right, you may have to purchase a forward seatpost and/or a shorter or longer front stem. A retailer can advise you if you come to this crossroads. Note that some manufacturers make adjustable stems. These are a worthy investment, because they allow you to more easily adjust your riding position to suit circumstances.

You can also adjust the tilt of your aerobar and, on many models, the separation of the elbow pads. The pads should be as close together as comfort allows, and the aero bar tilt should place your forearms either parallel to the top tube or angled slightly upward. Personal preference prevails in making these final adjustments. For that matter, personal preference should prevail with respect to the *entire* aero position. I'm just telling you what the pros tend to do, and what wind tunnel tests recommend. But the final step in the setup process should always be to get on the bike and ride, and if something doesn't feel right, by all means, adjust it away from the norm. Each rider is unique.

If you ride a road bike without an aerobar, use the following test to set the saddle setback position (and possibly also the front stem length): Mount the bike and place your hands on the brake hoods as you would when riding. In the ideal position for maximum power production (for most people), the middle section of the handlebar should completely obstruct your view of the front wheel hub. (The hub should be partially visible *behind* the handlebar when your hands are placed on the handlebar tops and should be visible *in front of* the handlebar when your hands are placed in the handlebar drops.) Make the saddle adjustments needed to pass this test. You should feel fairly open in this position, but not overly stretched. Keep in mind that moving the saddle back also increases the distance between your hips and the pedals, so if you find that you have to move the saddle way back in order to achieve a good road riding posture, you may need to go with a longer stem.

To really dial in the position, you can perform another test. Either install a power meter (such as an SRM or PowerTap) on your bike or mount your bike on an indoor trainer/ergometer that allows you to measure your power output (watts). Strap on a heart rate monitor as well (some ergometers come with built-in heart rate sensors). After a good warm-up, choose a moderate heart rate, hold it steady, and note your power output. Dismount, and make any desired adjustment to one of your bike settings. Repeat the test and note whether your power output increases or decreases at a consistent heart rate. Continue fiddling and tweaking (perhaps over a period of several days, as fatigue will raise your heart rate and skew results) until you've found your maximum power output riding position, which should also feel quite comfortable. You can perform this test for the aero riding position, too, but keep in mind that the ideal aero position is never the most powerful position, as aerodynamics and power output tend to work at cross purposes. Here, you just want to make sure you're not losing *too much power* for the sake of minimizing drag.

Pedaling and Cadence

The two components of pedaling are technique and cadence. Despite the expression "It's like riding a bike," proper pedaling technique and cadence often do not come naturally and require long practice to cultivate. The three characteristics of good pedaling technique are immobility above the hips (except when pedaling out of the saddle), no lateral movement of the legs or feet, and a relatively even application of force throughout the pedal stroke. The three most common errors in pedaling technique are body rocking, wide knees, and pedal stomping.

Rocking in the saddle is a waste of energy. Its most common causes are lack of sufficient flexibility in the hamstrings and hip flexors, weakness in the gluteal muscles, having the saddle positioned too high, and riding in too high a gear. If you find that you do tend to rock in the saddle, first of all check your seat height and your pedaling cadence. Failure to maintain a pedaling cadence of at least 70 revolutions per minute on all terrain except steep climbs and descents is an indication that your gear selection is poor. But if you can eliminate these causes, you should concentrate on correcting muscular imbalances in your lower body through stretching and functional strength training (see Chapter 8). Complement these measures with kinesthetic awareness, by which I mean paying attention to your form when you ride and consciously not rocking in the saddle.

The problem of wide knees is caused by the above-mentioned muscular imbalances, typically, and is often exacerbated by setting the saddle low, which many cyclists do because of their muscular imbalances (especially tight hamstrings). To correct wide knees, first check your bike setup; if it seems right, or if you cannot comfortably pedal in the correct position, begin to work on improving the elasticity of your hamstrings. As your flexibility improves, you should find that you can (and must) readjust your bike setup (possibly including your cleat position). Also, as with hip rocking, you should pay attention to your form when riding and force those knees in when you catch them creeping wide

Pedal stomping—also called mashing—is a descriptive term for failure to apply force evenly throughout the pedal stroke. In particular, it entails concentrating force on the downward, gravity-assisted portion of the pedal stroke and allowing momentum to carry the pedal back around to the top. Beyond the gravity factor, the reason this problem is so common is that the muscles that serve as the prime movers for the upward half of the pedal stroke, the hip extensors (gluteals and hamstrings), are relatively weak and underdeveloped in the average citizen because of all the sitting we do. The longer you continue to pedal stomp, the more pronounced the imbalance that caused you to stomp in the first place will become.

Analysis of world-class cyclists indicates that torque is maximized throughout the pedal stroke when hip and knee flexion and extension are finely coordinated with ankle flexion and extension. In the twelve o'clock to three o'clock portion of the pedal stroke, the hip and knee extend and the ankle flexes (heel comes down) so that force is generated both forward and downward, as the pedal is indeed moving both downward and forward during this portion of the stroke. From three o'clock to six o'clock, the hip and knee continue to extend as the ankle returns to neutral and begins to extend (toes go down), so that force is applied first straight downward, then downward and backward, in keeping with the motion of the pedal. Between six o'clock and nine o'clock, the hip and knee flex as the ankle extends sharply (heel comes up). Imagine that you're trying to kick yourself in the butt with your own heel. The sensation should be one of pulling *back* rather than upward. Although counterintuitive for many cyclists, this is actually the most effective way to make the pedal move upward from the bottom of the rotation. From nine o'clock back to twelve o'clock, as the hip and the knee continue to flex, the ankle returns to neutral. This final portion of the stroke is sometimes referred to as the "dead spot," even for those with perfect technique, because you're not really applying directional force here but rather keeping the weight of your foot and leg off the pedal in order to allow it to move unhindered, because by this time your other foot is pushing straight down on the opposite pedal, and this is the most powerful portion of the stroke.

You won't master this pattern just by thinking about it. You need to learn it by feel. There are a few good indoor cycling drills that can help you develop this feel. The best time to practice these methods is during the off-season transition period of training and the early portion of the base phase, when we tend to be indoors more, anyway, and we aren't so worried about fitness! fitness! fitness! Here they are:

Riding on Rollers

Mount your bike on indoor rollers and do a normal training ride. If your pedal stroke is uneven, the whirring sound made by the friction between your rear tire and the rollers will also sound uneven. By striving for an even whir, you will learn what good technique feels like as well as practice it.

Single-Leg Pedaling

Mount your bike on a wind trainer or simply seat yourself on a stationary bike. Pedal in a low gear (low resistance level) with a single leg while keeping your other leg out of the way (on a chair). Go for one minute, and then switch legs. Repeat the drill a few times more. Any stroke inconsistencies will be greatly exaggerated, as you won't have the other foot stomping while the one is supposed to be pulling. By striving for a fluid motion, you will once again learn what good technique feels like while grooving it.

Spin Scanning

Mount your bike on a wind trainer and hook it up to software that gives you a graphic display of your stroke on a television screen, as CompuTrainer's SpinScan does. While doing any kind of indoor training ride, you can learn and practice good technique by trying to make your stroke look right.

Spinning Out

Yet another way to improve pedaling technique is with a drill called spinning out, which involves gradually increasing your pedaling cadence over the course of several minutes, in a very low gear, until you reach maximum RPM, which you then maintain for 30 to 60 seconds. In this drill, stroke imbalances will reveal themselves in causing your rear end to bounce, which you must therefore try to prevent. Spinning out is best performed on an indoor trainer as well.

Pedaling cadence is a more individual matter. Here's why. Weight and drag held constant, how fast you travel on your bike is purely a matter of how much power you generate through the pedaling motion. As indicated above, your power output is a function of your gear selection (high or low) and your pedaling cadence (fast or slow). It is possible, therefore, to achieve any given power output in more than one way. For example, to maintain a power output of X, you might pedal rather slowly in a very high gear, pedal pretty fast in a slightly lower gear, or pedal really fast in a still lower gear. However, it's not all the same, because in one of these gear-cadence combinations you will be using the least amount of energy to produce the same amount of power. This combination is simply better suited to your body's way of generating power on a bicycle. At higher power output levels, most cyclists pedal with the greatest efficiency in the range of 75 to 90 RPM.

The hitch is that cyclists very often do not naturally pedal within their range of greatest efficiency. Put another way, for a majority of less experienced cyclists and even many veteran cyclists, *natural cadence* does not match *optimal cadence*. (The tendency is to pedal too slowly in too high a gear.) Because relatively few cyclists discover their optimal cadence by instinct, it's a good idea to look for it, so that you can work on bringing together your natural and optimal cadences. There's a high-tech way and a low-tech way do this. The high-tech way requires the use of a bike computer that allows you to track cadence, power output, and heart rate simultaneously. Use this device for most or all of your training and watch the interplay of these three variables in a variety of circumstances while playing with various gear-cadence combinations. What you're looking for is the cadence that's associated with the lowest heart rate at any single power output level in each situation, where situations are distinguished mainly by the terrain (flats versus various gradients) and by the level of intensity you wish to maintain.

This procedure will give you information about which gear to choose and cadence to adopt in every scenario. For example, former pro triathlete Jimmy Riccitello began studying his cadence rather late in his career and discovered, among other things, that he should always stay seated and raise his cadence to 100 RPM on medium-length steep hills, whereas it had always been his habit previously to get out of the saddle in such circumstances.

If you like to take a more carefree approach to your training, there's another way to bring together your optimal cadence and your natural cadence. As I mentioned above, power output on the bike is a function of gear selection and pedaling cadence. For this reason, every cyclist should train toward being able to push higher gears and maintain higher cadences. In other words, you should devote a portion of your training to pushing higher gears than you're comfortable pushing and maintaining higher cadences than you're used to maintaining (called spinning). I recommend spinning through a majority of your rides during the first several weeks of the base phase and performing one shorter training ride per week during the second half of the base phase in which you purposely pedal in high gears, at a sub-optimal cadence. You can also combine spinning and high-gear riding within a single Cadence Workout as described below. Reaching beyond your comfort zone in these ways will automatically tend to close any existing gap between your preferred and optimal cadences, even if you never bother to quantify your optimal cadence (which you're trying to change, anyway).

Other Bike Skills

Beyond pedaling technique and cadence, there are two additional bike skill categories whose elements you should master for the sake of safety and performance. The first of these two categories is riding in what we might call special circumstances. The particular skills within this category include climbing, descending, and cornering. The second category of skills is bicycle maintenance and upkeep.

Climbing

Good climbing starts with knowing how to read hills. Inexperienced cyclists often attack long hills too aggressively and "bonk" before they reach the top, or miss opportunities to use momentum against short, steep hills. Experienced cyclists know the best way to get up and over each hill based on familiarity with various hill types and knowledge of their personal climbing style. If you lack this ability, you will acquire it rapidly simply by taking on lots of hills in training and paying attention when you do.

On gradual hills, you can ride more or less the same way you do on the flats (only not as fast, of course). On tougher hills, the game changes. Aerodynamics cease to matter as power output becomes paramount. But hill gradients change the position of your body in relation to your bike, so the best power positions for climbing are not the same as the best power position on the flats. On most short climbs, you should get out of the saddle and grind your way over in a standing position. This technique allows you to make the best use of the momentum you have upon reaching the hill. On longer climbs, you should stay seated but slide back on your saddle and place your hands on the handlebar tops, standing only occasionally, as a means of giving your "sitting" muscles a short break and of accelerating to crest hills. Smaller cyclists are generally better served to climb almost exclusively in the seated position, while larger and more powerful cyclists can get away with standing a little more. When beginning a climb, unless the hill is extremely abrupt, downshift one gear at a time in order to maintain your cadence and not to waste the momentum you gathered on the preceding flat or descent. This way you'll have gotten a good start on the hill by the time you've slowed to the speed at which you'll finish it.

Descending

The main factors that promote speedy descending are aerodynamics and a little fearlessness, but not in that order. The best downhill cyclists are always those who love speed and naturally feel in control at high speeds. The only thing these riders need to be taught is some technique—and, sometimes, a little rational restraint. On the other hand, cyclists who are made anxious by high-speed descending face the tougher task of learning to let go somewhat. This can be done gradually. One way to proceed is to ride the steepest descent on your favorite hilly training ride as slowly as you please, noting the highest speed you reach on your bike computer, and then try to beat this mark by just one mile per hour on each subsequent ride until your descending is no longer a liability.

As for technique, when starting a descent, just allow gravity to accelerate your bike as you maintain a consistent effort level. Shift up gradually to hold cadence steady until (supposing the descent is long and steep enough) you reach optimal cadence in your highest gear, at which time you should cease pedaling and hold your most aerodynamic riding position as you enjoy a simultaneous adrenaline rush and cardiovascular rest. If you have an aerobar, use it, unless there's any chance you'll need to break or turn suddenly. In that case, or if you lack an aerobar, place your hands in the handlebar drops, raise your butt several inches above your seat, and bring your knees toward each other. Resume pedaling whenever you feel yourself slowing. When coming off the descent, shift down gradually in order to make the best use of your momentum.

Cornering

Cornering is another skill that can require some derring-do, especially when combined with descending. This is because, at higher speeds, you do not make turns by turning your wheel but rather by *leaning*. The faster you wish to corner, and the sharper the turn, the more lean is required. Judging accurately how fast you can safely take a corner and how sharply you must lean in taking it are abilities that only experience can teach. If you must decelerate, always brake *before* you enter the turn, as braking while turning is inherently unstable (something to do with vector forces). Also, you should pedal only in long, sweeping turns. In tighter turns, make sure to cease pedaling with the inside pedal at the top of its rotation so it doesn't scuff the road, and for better balance. In races and rides wherein opposing traffic is not an issue, start wide and come in or start inside and come wide (depending on which side of the road you wish to end up on) in order to reduce the severity of your turn. And last, if the turn does result in significant loss of speed, stand up for several pedal strokes and sprint back to speed immediately upon coming out of the turn.

Maintenance and Upkeep

I like to think of the matter of bicycle maintenance and upkeep as having three tiers. The first tier is roadside repair. The second tier is regular upkeep. The third tier is the annual (or semiannual) overhaul. For roadside repair, always ride with a saddle pouch containing a spare tube, a patch kit, tire levers, a multitool containing 4-millimeter, 5-millimeter, and 6-millimeter hex wrenches, CO_2 cartridges (unless you happen to use a frame pump as your tire pressure source), and $20 in case of disaster. Know how to change a flat. Learn also how to diagnose the cause of each flat. There are three categories: punctures, characterized by a hole on the outside of the tube; pinch flats, characterized by a pair of holes; and flats caused by the tire rim itself, or by a foreign object inside the tire, which are characterized by a hole on the inside of the tube. Flats are by far the most common mid-ride mishap. The next most common showstopper is when things (pedals, handlebars, and so forth) come

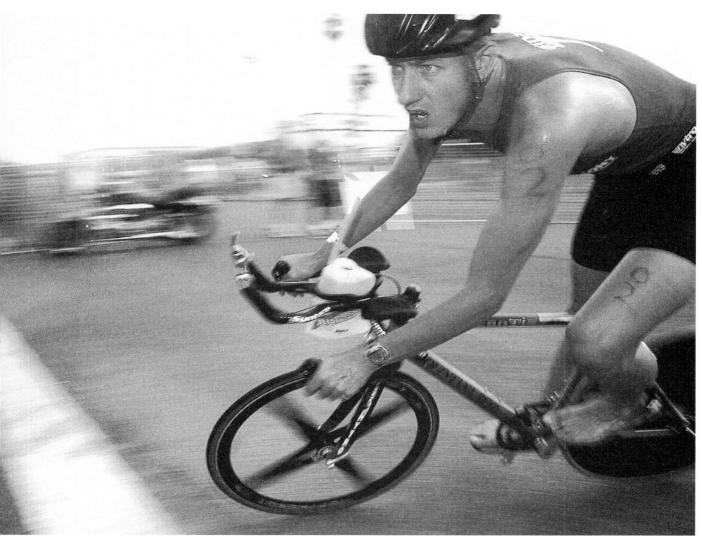

Good cornering skills can yield big time savings in races. *Robert Oliver*

loose, which is why you need the multitool and knowledge of how to use it. After that, it's broken chains, which require a special tool and just a smidgen of know-how to fix. I carry a chain tool on my longest rides only. Each of these skills is best learned hands-on from a fellow cyclist or from one of the many bike mechanics who offer basic repair classes out of their shops.

Before each ride, you should check the pressure of your tires and inflate them if necessary and perform a two-minute safety check, making sure your spokes have tension, your handlebar and/or aerobar doesn't slip when pushed, your chain is properly lubricated, and your wheels are trued and clamped on correctly. Loose bolts and such you can fix yourself. For jobs like wheel truing and spoke retensioning, you'll need professional assistance. Lubricate your chain every 100 miles or so. Keep an eye on tire wear as well. A high-quality pair of training tires will typically last 1,500 miles or so (the front tire always wears out first). Check the tension on your derailleur cables, too, and know how to adjust them if there's any slack (another skill you can quickly pick up from a more experienced cyclist). Always clean and lube your bike before races, tighten bolts, install your racing tires, and inflate them at the last minute. If you travel by plane with your bike, to races or other events, proper use of most bike cases requires that you be comfortable removing and replacing your wheels, pedals, and handlebar.

Once a year—or twice a year, if you do mega-mileage—take your bike to the best shop in your area for a professional overhaul. This service will cost you in the range of $120 to $160, but will more than pay for itself in the form of performance and longevity. Choose your bike mechanic as carefully as you would (or should) choose an automobile mechanic, especially if you have high-end equipment on your bike. I'm sorry to say that many mechanics take little pride in their work, and just as many are marginally competent, or less. The overhaul will entail complete disassembly of your bike, a thorough cleaning, inspection of all parts, diagnosis of wear and failure, rebuilding, and recommended replacements. Brake pads and drive train components (chain, freewheel, etc.) are the most common replacements required. In addition to necessary replacements, this is a perfect time to make any upgrades you've planned.

Cycling Workouts

The key to performing appropriate cycling workouts is mastering intensity. This entails, first of all, emphasizing the right intensities in the right proportions in the right sequence, and second, actually performing your workouts at the intended intensity levels. Controlling intensity on the bike can be somewhat trickier than doing so in the pool because the open roads represent a less controlled environment. But it's not rocket science either.

The two levels of training intensity that are simultaneously the most difficult and most important to find exactly are threshold and max oxygen intensity, as these intensities correspond with precise physiological thresholds. The best way to ensure that you actually do train at these intensities when you want to is by perceived effort, in the context of appropriately structured workouts. Threshold pace feels comfortable, but just barely. You should perform threshold workouts at the fastest pace that feels more or less comfortable the whole way through. For athletes with a fitness base, threshold pace is the fastest pace that can be maintained for about an hour of cycling. A good threshold workout, therefore, is to ride 20 to 40 minutes (depending on your fitness level) at a pace you feel you could maintain for 60 minutes and no more in race circumstances. In the final minutes of a threshold workout, you should feel the first hints of fatigue but little or no lactic acid burn in your legs.

Max oxygen pace is the fastest pace a cyclist with a solid fitness base can maintain for about 15 minutes. You know you're working at max oxygen intensity when you can feel that you've reached your maximum capacity for controlled breathing. A good max oxygen workout is four to eight intervals lasting four to five minutes each and ridden at a pace you feel you could maintain for no more than about 15 minutes. If you reach the state of maximum respiration less than a minute or so into each interval, you're going too fast (or you haven't rested enough). If you feel you could inhale and exhale a little harder without hyperventilating, you're going too easy. Also, if you perform your max oxygen workouts correctly, your last interval should be performed at the same pace as your first, and you should be quite sure that you could complete at most one more interval at the same pace, and possibly none at all.

You can enhance your mastery of bike training intensity by using the objective measurement of pace, heart rate, and power output. Simply do your workouts using a cyclometer, heart rate monitor, and/or an SRM or PowerTap and note the readings they give you as you train. You can then use these devices over time to track your fitness progress, adjust to unfamiliar courses, and (in the case of pace measurement) set race goals. Just keep in mind that terrain and environmental conditions affect pace, while these and a host of other conditions can affect heart rate. Power output is more constant, but of course it will gradually increase in relation to any given training intensity as your fitness increases, so perceived effort must always have the final say.

How about the other intensities? Endurance intensity is simply anything below threshold level and above recovery level. Most of your endurance training should be performed near the middle of this broad range, well above recovery intensity and well below threshold intensity. Recovery intensity corresponds more or less to the threshold where carbohydrate burning eclipses fat burning, but you certainly can't feel this threshold in the way you can feel lactic acid buildup or maximum respiration, and you'll do fine simply to make your recovery training feel very easy while still being intense enough to qualify as exercise. Your speed pace need not be precise, either. It can range from a pace just slightly faster than max oxygen pace to a full sprint, as long as it's done in an appropriate workout context. A good speed workout might consist of six to twelve intervals (depending on your fitness level) lasting 90 seconds each and separated by three or four minutes of recovery riding. Your pacing is appropriate if you complete the last interval at the same pace as your first and you feel you could perform no more than one additional interval at the same pace. Following are descriptions of workouts appropriate for every specific training effect. The most appropriate phases for each workout are indicated between parentheses.

RECOVERY RIDE

(BUILD, PEAK)

While there's no such thing as a recovery ride for triathletes who are just starting, or starting over, spinning easily for 20 minutes to an hour (and avoiding hills) is a great way to hasten the recovery process following races or hard workouts for those who have a high level of aerobic fitness.

ENDURANCE RIDE

(BASE, BUILD, PEAK)

The purpose of endurance rides is to develop the body's ability to consume oxygen and its ability to conserve carbohydrate fuel and thereby prolong endurance. They represent the very foundation of bike training. If you were to perform only one type of cycling workout, this would be it.

Endurance rides may take place at any intensity level, or any mix of intensities, below the threshold level. Duration can also vary widely. A typical endurance ride for a beginner should last about 40 minutes, while a typical endurance ride for a competitive triathlete training for a long-distance peak race should exceed two hours by the late base phase. Spinning is a type of endurance ride wherein one consciously maintains a high cadence (85–95 RPM) in an effort to gradually increase one's optimal cadence.

LONG RIDE

(BASE, BUILD, PEAK)

Beginning around the middle of the base phase, you should perform a weekly or biweekly long ride at endurance intensity that is significantly longer than any other endurance ride performed during the week. For triathletes training for longer races, and for triathletes for whom just finishing an upcoming race is the main challenge, these rides should reach their peak duration two to three weeks before the race. In other cases, they can peak at the end of the base phase and then be held constant for the remainder of the training cycle.

HARD GROUP RIDE

(BASE, BUILD, PEAK)

Hard group rides are more of a practical reality than a theoretical necessity. When you train with a group, which is good to do, you generally ride harder than when you ride alone. This is okay, to a point. Just make sure you do most of the ride below threshold intensity if it's intended as an endurance ride, and that it fits the formats preferable for high-intensity rides if it's intended as a high-intensity ride.

THRESHOLD RIDE

(BUILD, PEAK)

In the middle of an otherwise endurance-intensity ride, cycle 20 to 40 minutes at or near threshold intensity on flat or mostly flat terrain. Do shorter threshold rides earlier in the training cycle and increase their duration slightly in each subsequent ride.

LONG HILL REPEATS

(BUILD)

After completing a thorough warm-up, do four to eight climbs lasting four to five minutes each on a moderately steep hill. Stay seated throughout the climbs and make sure your effort level does not creep above your VO_2 max threshold. Keep your cadence at or above 60 RPM, and select your gear accordingly. Take three or four minutes of active recovery between climbs. Finish with a thorough cool-down. To avoid coasting downhill between climbs, or if you live in a flat area, you can perform this workout on an indoor cycling ergometer with simulated climbs.

SHORT HILL REPEATS

(BUILD)

This is a speed-intensity workout. Following a long warm-up, do six to 12 climbs lasting roughly 90 seconds each on a fairly steep hill. Do the first two thirds of each climb seated and stand for the final push. The intensity is too high if you're not able to make each climb as fast as, or slightly faster than, the previous. Finish with a thorough cool-down. Again, to avoid coasting downhill between climbs, or if you live in a flat area, you can perform this workout on an indoor cycling ergometer with simulated climbs.

TIME TRIAL

(BUILD, PEAK)

Warm up thoroughly and then ride between 10K and 10 miles (a distance you can complete in about 20 minutes) at maximum effort, which will correspond approximately to max oxygen intensity. If possible, do this workout on a marked course, or simply find landmarks at the start and finish points, so that you can come back to it and gauge your progress. Cool down long and easy.

CADENCE WORKOUT

(PRE-BASE, BASE)

After warming up, ride for 20 to 40 minutes at the high end of endurance intensity while alternating between three-minute bouts at 70 RPM and three-minute bouts at 90–100 RPM. Try to keep your heart rate constant and select your gears accordingly. Finish with a nice, long cool-down. This workout will help to increase your optimal cadence and your power output.

POWER INTERVALS (SPRINTS)

(BASE, BUILD)

During an endurance-intensity ride, do four to 10 sprints lasting roughly 30 seconds each. Accelerate to maximum speed out of the saddle and then sit for the remainder of the sprint. The purpose of

Recommended Bike Training Parameters

The table below suggests basic bike training parameters for triathletes in each of four very general categories. Note the broad recommended weekly mileage ranges. These reflect two considerations: the necessary volume ramp-up that must occur in the base phase and the broad range of competitive ambitions with which individual triathletes approach triathlons of the same length.

Category			Base Phase	Build Phase	Peak Phase
Beginner	Key Workouts		Endurance	Endurance	Brick
	Weekly Mileage		12–20	15–25	20–35
Sprint	Key Workouts		Endurance	Max Oxygen, Speed, Brick	Threshold, Brick
	Weekly Mileage		30–100	40–100	40–100
Middle	Key Workouts		Endurance	Max Oxygen, Brick, Speed	Threshold, Long Ride, Brick
	Weekly Mileage		40–150	60–150	60–200
Long	Key Workouts		Endurance, Long Ride, Brick	Threshold, Long Ride, Brick, Max Oxygen	Long Ride, Brick
	Weekly Mileage		80–250	100–250	120–300

Table 4.1

this workout, as the name suggests, is to increase your muscle power. Recover for several minutes after each hard effort. When performed in the context of group rides, such sprints are known as *jumps*.

INDOOR GROUP RIDE

(PRE-BASE, BASE)

If you belong to a fitness club that offers group cycling workouts, you may wish to participate in them every now and again, especially during the winter, for a change of pace. The music, social atmosphere, and high intensity make them enjoyable and fruitful, even if they don't yield any specific training effect, as intensity is all over the place.

BRICK

(BASE, BUILD, PEAK)

A *brick* workout is (usually) a bike ride followed immediately by a run, and it's a type of workout that is unique to triathlon (and duathlon). There are many ways to approach a brick. I recommend doing one brick each week throughout most of the training cycle and varying the approach based on your location within the cycle. For example, during the late base phase you might do a moderately long ride followed by a moderately long run, both at endurance intensity. In the early peak phase, you might do a threshold ride followed by a tempo run. Feel free to mix it up, so long as the intensity of the two segments makes sense in terms of your present training needs and you make sure to count a high-intensity brick against the total number of high-intensity workouts you can handle in one week.

Periodization of Bike Training

Following is a concise characterization of the best way to approach your bike training in each of the three main phases of the training cycle. In Chapter 6 I'll talk about how to mix together swim, bike, and run training in all three phases.

Base

Your primary goal during the base phase is to lay a broad foundation of aerobic capacity and raw endurance. Secondary emphases are improving technique and increasing cadence and pedaling power.

Begin the phase with low volume and low intensity and gradually increase both. At first, most workouts should take place in the lower end of the endurance intensity range. By the end of the phase, most workouts should take place in the middle and upper parts of this range, as in hard group rides. Throughout the phase, the majority of your endurance rides should entail spinning at a slightly higher than optimal pedaling cadence. Also in the first several weeks of the base phase, do one or two technique drills each week and a set of power intervals or jumps in one of your weekly endurance rides.

After a few weeks of base building, begin doing one weekly or biweekly long ride and increase the duration of this ride slightly every other week (whether you do it weekly or biweekly). About the same time, begin performing a weekly brick workout.

Toward the end of the base phase, mix in some more high-intensity training in an informal way. One way to do this is to begin attacking the hills you encounter in your endurance rides. Another way is by participating in indoor group cycling workout classes. Speaking of which, if all or part of your base phase coincides with winter, be prepared to do most or all of your cycling workouts indoors.

Build

In the build phase, your primary objective is to maximize your aerobic capacity by emphasizing above-threshold-intensity training. Start with a single, formal high-intensity ride per week and add a second one only if you're handling the first quite easily and have competitive ambitions.

My first recommendation is that you begin with a weekly speed-intensity workout such as short hill intervals, and after doing a few of these, switch over to weekly max-oxygen-intensity workouts, such as time trials, which are more taxing and more race-specific in their training effect. However, you can reverse the order if you wish, or alternate the two types, and still make similar gains in fitness. I myself like to alternate them, while doing the same in running, but on opposite weeks (for example, a speed run and a max oxygen ride this week, a max oxygen run and a speed ride next week). If you're doing two quality bike workouts a week, do a speed-pace ride and a max-oxygen-pace ride. Another option is to eschew speed-intensity workouts entirely and get what little speed-intensity training you need by continuing to perform power intervals or jumps within one or two of your weekly endurance rides. In this case, you'll want to introduce threshold-intensity rides where the speed-intensity rides might have taken place.

Your overall training volume should remain fairly consistent throughout this phase, but do continue to practice step cycles. Maintain the duration of your long rides as well. Keep doing weekly brick workouts. You may also begin doing lower-priority races during this phase.

Peak

Your main objective in the peak phase is to maximize race readiness by emphasizing race-specific workouts and getting adequate rest, especially toward the end of the phase. Perform one threshold-intensity ride per week throughout this phase, as this intensity level is close to race intensity for many triathletes in many races. In any event, it's closer than max oxygen and speed intensity. Perform a small amount of training at these higher intensity levels at your discretion. In addition to these threshold rides, you should do a ride at precisely your goal race pace at least every other week throughout the peak phase.

If your final peak race is a long-distance event, or an event that will be challenging just to finish, your training volume and the duration of your long rides should begin once again to steadily increase in this phase. Otherwise, they should be held steady. Continue doing that weekly brick workout. Also, in this phase be sure to do at least one or two (short- or middle-distance) triathlons prior to the peak triathlon that falls at the end of the phase, and of the training cycle as a whole. These races will both reward and increase your fitness.

Within a week to three weeks of your final peak triathlon, it's time to taper. Cut out the long rides and reduce total bike training volume incrementally. Maintain the intensity of your quality workouts, but reduce the volume here as well.

Being a Triathlon Fan

Triathlon is primarily a participatory sport, but it is also a professional sport. I find that being a fan of professional triathlon adds an enjoyable dimension to my experience as a triathlon participant, and I reckon it can do the same for any triathlete. Watching world-class athletes compete is pleasurable, inspirational, and sometimes even educational. And as with any other sport, rooting for your favorite athletes or for athletes representing your nation can be wonderfully exciting (though sometimes heartbreaking, too!).

But because triathlon is not a major spectator sport like baseball and leapfrog, enjoying professional competition is not as easy as turning on the television and watching this weekend's most important race as it unfolds. It takes a little savvy to be a triathlon fan. Here are my recommendations.

Pardon my partiality, but the best place to start is with *Triathlete* magazine. By reading *Triathlete* (and, if you must, another triathlon monthly), you will quickly become familiar with the major events and the names, looks, and personalities of the best professional athletes. In-depth race reports help you appreciate what it takes to win at the highest levels and high-quality action photography captures the beauty of championship form.

The Internet satisfies the triathlon fan's needs on a more frequent and faster basis. In addition to *Triathlete*'s Web site (www.triathletemag.com), several other fine triathlon Web sites provide breaking news, race previews, race results, and sometimes even live event coverage. For example, Ironmanlive.com provides real-time coverage of several Ironman triathlons that gets better and more sophisticated each year. I log into each of three or four different triathlon Web sites a few times each week.

As for television, my first recommendation is that you move to Australia. There are no bigger triathlon fans than the Aussies, who are rewarded for their enthusiasm with the privilege of being able to watch their country's thrilling Formula One events and other big races live on national television, start to finish. In other countries, however, the pickings are slim. In the United States, several Ironman events are broadcast as one-hour specials (two hours for Hawaii) on networks like ESPN and NBC, but way after the fact. Only a smattering of other triathlons receive television airtime (among them, Escape from Alcatraz, Mrs. T's Chicago), but again, always edited and after the fact, and sometimes only locally. Still, such programs have their value for fanatics. For example, I'll never forget the thrill of tuning in to see Belgium's Luc Van Lierde record the fastest Ironman time in history at the 1997 Ironman Europe, even though I had learned of the performance weeks beforehand.

But nothing beats watching world-class triathlon competition in person. Fortunately, the directors of many larger triathlons kindly separate their age group and pro waves by sufficient time to allow the age-groupers to complete their race and hang out to watch the elites go at it. I recommend taking advantage of this opportunity whenever possible, even to the point of selecting events that attract strong pro fields over other race options that do not. And, of course, there's nothing stopping you from showing up just to watch races that happen to take place in your area, as I sometimes do.

There's even one triathlon I would recommend traveling just to see: the hallowed Hawaii Ironman, which takes place each year on the first Saturday after the first full moon in October in Kailua Kona, Hawaii. Make a week of it, taking in all the Super Bowl–like hoopla that precedes the race itself, including the parade, press conference, autograph signings, pro bike check-in, and final swims at Dig-Me Beach. The race itself is one of the most awesome spectacles you'll ever see: the world's finest endurance specimens reaching deeper than one would think possible to overcome fierce rivals and fiercer conditions for glory and not much money. Oh, and the Olympics. I would also condone traveling anywhere in the world except maybe Beijing to see the Olympic Triathlons.

Finally, any fan of triathlon might as well be a fan of the related sports of swimming, running, track and field, cycling, and mountain biking. It's that much more material for enjoyment, inspiration, and learning. Just be sure you're not watching when you ought to be doing!

CHAPTER 5

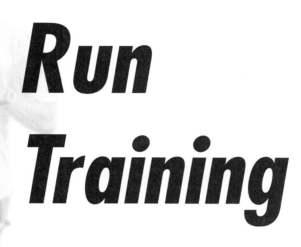

Run Training

And then there's running. What's running all about? If you pose this question to the average citizen, who knows nothing about the sport of long-distance running, and who probably loathes the activity, he or she will likely tell you that running is all about being skinny. And that's not far from the truth. Much more so than it is to the swimmer or the cyclist, body weight is to runners what kryptonite is to Superman. Worse than useless, it's totally counterproductive. Rare is the champion male marathoner who weighs more than 150 pounds, and physiology tells us why. A runner weighing 160 pounds burns about 6.5 percent more energy than a runner weighing 150 pounds and maintaining the same pace.

Yet not every skinny person is a good runner, nor is every good runner skinny. (A friend of mine ran a 2:28 marathon at 187 pounds.) This is because there's a slight difference between *being* skinny and *running* skinny. You see, body weight is not inherently bad for the runner, but only bad inasmuch as it increases the energy demands of running. Yet there are other factors beyond body weight that influence the relative energy demands of running. Running form and economy are the other major ones. And by making the most of these factors, even the tall and broad runner can learn to "run skinny." This is a good thing, because you can't replace the body you were given.

So, while good running is certainly assisted by the right genetically bestowed body type, any runner can improve significantly with proper training. The goal of this chapter is to show you how to train to run skinny, as it were.

The Nature of Run Training

Running is more intense, in the physiological sense of the word, than either swimming or cycling. The highest heart rate you can achieve while running is higher than the highest heart rate you can achieve while cycling, which is higher than the highest heart rate you can achieve while swimming. This is the case because running activates more muscle mass and entails greater gravitational resistance. Running is therefore more stressful than the other two triathlon disciplines. We simply cannot handle as much high-intensity running. Long-distance runners could never race every weekend as cyclists do, or do interval workouts several times a week like swimmers.

Moreover, due to the high-impact nature of running, we simply cannot handle as much running at *any* intensity level as we can handle swimming and cycling. The chances of incurring overuse injuries, and also the variety of injuries incurred, are far greater. Consequently, elite distance runners spend on average less than a quarter as much time training as elite swimmers and cyclists do, and still they get injured far more. Beyond limiting their training volume, runners of all levels must also vigilantly practice a variety of injury-prevention measures, including running off-road when possible, increasing volume very gradually, stretching, and treating incipient injuries the moment symptoms appear.

Another difference between run training and swim and bike training is the track factor. Most competitive runners visit a track facility for one or two high-intensity workouts a week, whereas most swimmers do all of their training in the pool and most cyclists do their low-intensity and high-intensity training on the same roads, except when weather forbids it. Running on the track is never completely necessary for triathletes, but there is much to be said for the controlled environment it affords, especially when it comes to training by pace. I myself love the track, but I'm aware that many triathletes can't stand running in tight circles, so while I do recommend that you make use of a track for most of your max oxygen and speed workouts, I won't insist on it!

The primary difference between single-sport running and triathlon running is that the latter always takes place in a fatigued state, immediately following at least 45 minutes and possibly as much as nine or ten hours of racing in the other two disciplines. Triathletes prepare for fatigued running primarily by practicing it in brick workouts, but also simply by training for a higher level of raw endurance than runners, which is a natural consequence of training in three endurance disci-

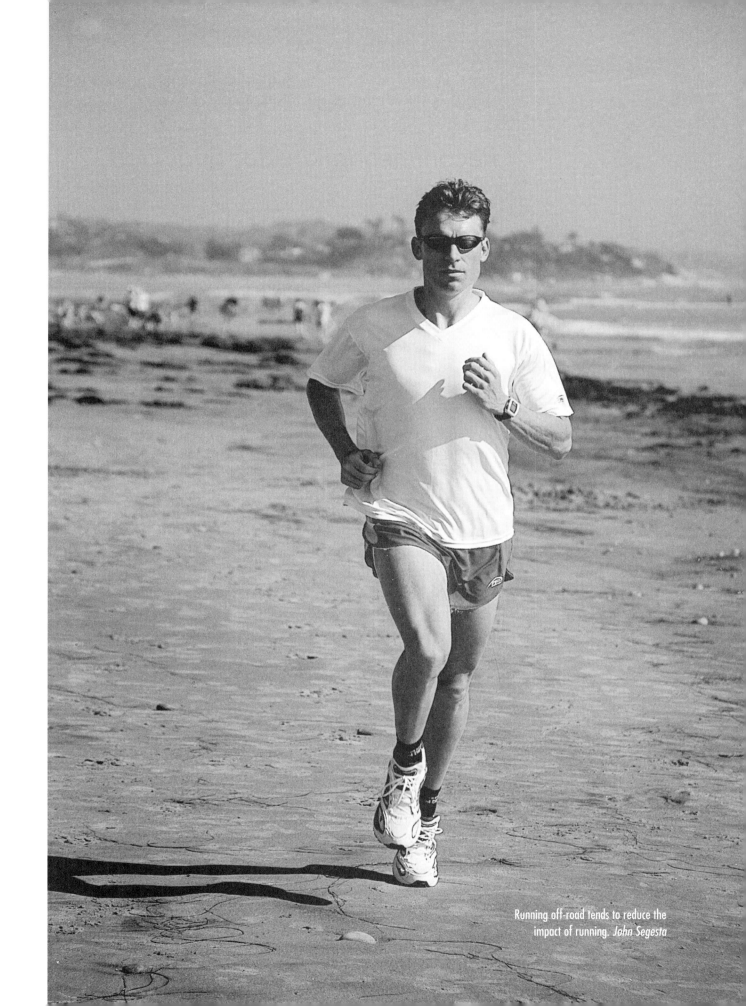

Running off-road tends to reduce the impact of running. *John Segesta*

plines. In other words, triathletes train for running by swimming and cycling, as well as running, and relying upon a crossover effect.

Recommendations for Beginners

Running is not the kind of activity one jumps into with both feet, so to speak, especially as an adult. If you are currently a nonrunner, my advice is that you begin with a few weeks of walk-run workouts, preferably on softer surfaces, before you graduate to normal running workouts. While you may have the endurance needed to run for 20 or 30 minutes consecutively, the tissues of your lower extremities will almost certainly lack the durability to survive a sudden habituation to repetitive impact without breaking down very quickly. Various overuse injuries, including iliotibial band syndrome, runner's knee, shin splints, Achilles tendinitis, and plantar fasciitis (all discussed in Chapter 8), commonly befall triathletes and runners who ramp up their running volume too quickly.

Begin with 20 or 30 minutes of brisk walking on a track or packed dirt trail with two or three two-minute jogging intervals tossed in. Don't panic about fitness. You're still swimming and cycling, and even brisk walking provides a good workout for a relative beginner. Gradually increase the duration of your jogging intervals from one workout to the next until you're jogging straight through. Only then, and again, only gradually, should you transition to pavement. But don't ever feel compelled to run on roads. In fact, the more total running you do, the greater the fraction of it you should do off-road, if possible.

If you're overweight, it's especially important that you proceed with caution in your run training. In fact, it's not a bad idea for those carrying a few extra pounds to swim and cycle *only* until they've trimmed down, and then engage in the above walk-run progression.

I recommend this approach even to those who have done a lot of running in the past, but none recently. It's all the same. I know this from experience. A competitive runner in my youth, I hung up my shoes for a few years before the lure of triathlon inspired me to begin pounding (and I do mean pounding) the pavement once more. Forgetting the passage of time, I ramped up my mileage too quickly, developed shin splints, and was forced to start over.

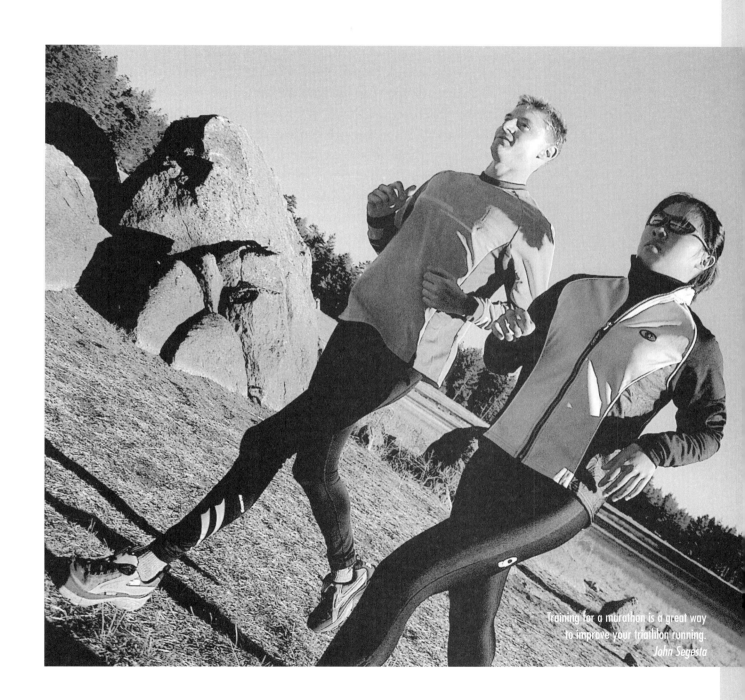

Training for a marathon is a great way
to improve your triathlon running.
John Segesta

Running Form

The good news is that good running form is not complicated. On the contrary, it could scarcely be simpler. The bad news is that good running form is rare and also difficult to teach or learn. To a far greater degree than swimming and pedaling technique, good running form is the kind of thing you either have, or you don't. By the time children are eight or nine years old you can tell who the potentially talented distance runners are by observing their natural, uncoached stride. They're the lucky ones. But you *can* improve your running form—you just can't do so quite as straightforwardly as you can improve swimming or pedaling technique.

There are three effective methods of improving running technique. The first is running fast. Running form tends naturally to become more efficient as intensity increases. By performing an adequate amount of running at the max-oxygen intensity level and especially the speed intensity level, you can become a more efficient runner generally. A second means of improving running technique is by achieving better muscular balance through functional strength training, stretching, and technique drills like hill bounding. Muscular imbalances contribute to inefficiencies in running and also to the many injuries that can result from them. A third method of improving running form is through the practice of kinesthetic awareness—that is, through consciously correcting your form during the act of running. This practice requires patience and perseverance to succeed, and in most instances it must also be accompanied by efforts to remedy muscular imbalances.

As with swimming and cycling, good running form is all about maximizing efficiency and power. There are six basic characteristics of good running form: high stride rate, minimal ground contact, long strides, high kick, relaxed upper body, and symmetry. Each of these six characteristics is associated with either efficiency or power, or both. Let's take a look at the components of good running form and how to develop each.

High Stride Rate

Good running form is characterized first of all by a high stride rate. The best runners, male and female, tall and short, take 180 or more strides per minute when racing and only slightly fewer strides when running at lower intensity levels. Fast and slow runners alike increase stride length more than they do stride rate when increasing speed. It seems that each person has a natural stride rate, but unfortunately, not every natural stride rate is as good as every other. Again, faster is better.

In light of this reality, many running and triathlon coaches tell athletes to simply practice running with a faster stride rate—which also means shorter strides, if pace is held constant—in their training. I don't think this works. I've never seen it work, or known of any instance of its working, and there's no scientific evidence that it works either.

So, instead, I recommend running at high speeds as a much more natural way of practicing a higher stride rate. Even though stride length increases more than stride rate as your speed increases, stride rate does increase, and the fact is, you *will* take close to 180 strides per minute if you run fast enough. And if you run fast enough often enough, you will gain some efficiency at this rate and perhaps see your stride rate increase at lower intensities. In addition to your actual speed repetitions on the track (discussed below), you should perform four to six *strides* and/or *accelerations* after one or two weekly endurance runs throughout the year. A stride is simply 100 yards (or so) run at about one-mile race pace followed by a jogging recovery. An acceleration is 100 yards begun at your standard endurance pace and completed at a near sprint following a steady acceleration. Strides and accelerations can also be performed on hills and descents for variety and slightly different effects.

Minimal Ground Contact

Faster runners spend more time in the air and less time on the ground than slower runners. This only makes sense, because you're not moving forward when either foot is on the ground, but only between foot strikes. Also, the less time the foot spends on the ground, the quicker it applies force to the ground, and the more force the ground returns back to the foot for forward propulsion.

The major causes of longer foot strikes are striking heel first, lateral foot motion, and excessive vertical displacement, or "bouncing." Regarding the first of these, all runners push off with their toes. Therefore, the further away from your toes you land, the more time your foot spends on the ground as it rolls forward in preparation to push off. Studies have shown that only a small fraction of elite distance runners are heel strikers, while the majority are forefoot and midfoot strikers. Heel striking is caused by a tendency to reach out with the forward leg when running and place the foot down far ahead of one's center of gravity, which is bad not only because it results in more support time but also because it has a braking effect. Again, the solution to this error is not to force yourself to land on the midfoot or forefoot. Using kinesthetic awareness to modify your foot strike will be ineffective unless you do it in combination with other measures. The most effective such measure is, once more, to practice running fast, as there is a tendency to come forward on the foot at high speeds. In fact, nearly every runner is a forefoot striker when sprinting.

Performing downhill strides and accelerations is also helpful in this regard. Running downhill greatly increases the energy waste associated with heel striking. Of course, it becomes necessary to heel strike in order to control your speed and impact when you're on a steeper descent. But on a mild descent, when you wish to take advantage of gravity, you do so by pulling your center of gravity forward so that your feet land almost right underneath your body, and less on the heel. This is more or less how you want to run all the time, and performing strides or accelerations on a mild descent makes it profoundly obvious why you do and also gives you practice doing it.

Lateral motion of the foot also tends to increase the amount of time the foot spends on the ground during running and the amount of energy dissipation that occurs. The most common lateral motion problem is overpronation, which is a tendency of the foot to roll inward during the support phase. The opposite problem is oversupination. While not as common, it is equally detrimental from the standpoint of economy (and injury avoidance). If you suspect that you have a problem with lateral foot motion, you should wear running shoes designed to limit lateral motion, and you may need to purchase a pair of special insoles that are designed to correct your specific type of problem. There are many and sundry options available, so you may need to try a few different kinds before you find the one that works best. If your problem is severe, and especially if your problem is compounded by a very low or very high arch, you should see a podiatrist who understands running and have yourself fit for prescription orthotics inserts. But shoes, inserts, and orthotics only manage the problem of lateral foot motion and do not treat its root cause, which often includes some form of muscular imbalance.

The tendency to bounce when running is one of the easiest form deficiencies to unlearn, because it is generally caused by thinking *too much* about form (i.e., trying to look cute) when running. The surest way to get rid of it is to run far. When you're tired, you can no longer afford to waste the kind of energy you waste by bouncing. Running on sand also increases the price you pay for bouncing and therefore helps to eliminate it. And, of course, running fast works here, too.

Long Strides

Running speed is a function of stride rate and stride length. As indicated above, the factor that changes the most when running speed increases is stride length. From this it would seem to follow that being able to take longer strides is the key to faster running. But if this were true, the best distance runners would be tall, and this is seldom the case. Instead, the keys to faster running, as it relates to stride length, are generating power in the toe-off portion of the running stride and being able to take long strides *efficiently*.

The latter comes from plain old aerobic fitness. The more effectively your body consumes oxygen, the easier it becomes to sustain the level of energy output required to maintain any given stride length (pace). A powerful toe-off comes from strength in the calves, hamstrings, and feet. You can increase the strength of your leg muscles by performing the functional strength routines presented in Chapter 8. But a powerful push-off begins with your feet and ankles, and there are some easy ways to increase strength in these areas, too. One way is by laying a towel on the floor in front of your bare feet and using your toes to scrunch up the towel and pull it under your feet (you must be sitting for this to work). Picking up marbles with your toes repeatedly has a similar effect. And simply walking around barefoot as often as it's practical strengthens the feet as well.

There are also some ways to strengthen your feet and ankles within the context of your normal running workouts. An excellent example is hill bounding, which is basically what a triple jumper does in his or her first two jumps, except on an incline. It's an exaggerated running movement that results in greater than normal vertical and forward displacement. Do a few 100-yard stretches of hill bounding after the occasional endurance run, either mixed in with your strides and accelerations or in place of them. Running barefoot in sand is also an excellent means of developing stronger feet and ankles.

High Kick

Another component of good running form is a high kick, that is, lifting the foot high (up near the butt) during the recovery phase of the running stride. This results from bending the knee to an acute angle as soon as the push-off leg achieves full extension after toe-off, and it allows the runner to carry the recovery leg forward in a folded position that is much more energy efficient than dragging forward a straighter leg. Kick height is enhanced by stronger hamstrings, which in turn are achievable through functional strength training. Also, runners tend to kick higher as they run faster, so again, running fast is a good prescription to cure this form deficiency.

Relaxed Upper Body

The form of elite runners is often described as "effortless," and with good reason. Better runners do in fact use less energy to run at any given pace than average runners. In addition to the form components already mentioned, this efficiency comes from being able to relax the muscles that cannot contribute, or are not currently contributing, to forward movement. In particular, your upper body should be as relaxed as it can be without failing to contribute the necessary arm swing component of the running action.

Many runners and triathletes tense their upper bodies too much when running, especially at high intensities and high levels of fatigue. Teaching your upper body to relax sufficiently requires a consistent application of conscious effort at first. Put yourself in the habit of periodically focusing your attention on the muscles of your upper body when running, especially during quality workouts. When you discover that your shoulders are hunched, your fists are clenched, and the muscles in your arms are flexed, force them to relax. You may also try shaking out the arms periodically as a means of promoting upper body relaxation. While at first these measures may have only a very temporary effect that wears off as soon as your mental focus travels elsewhere, over time you can condition yourself to relax more generally despite fatigue and high intensity.

Symmetry

The significance of the fact that running is a one-leg-at-a-time activity is often overlooked. Any kind of imbalance between the left and right halves of the body can result in compensations that reduce economy (i.e., "skinniness") and lead to injury. Such imbalances are common. They can include leg length discrepancies, unequal strength in the left and right hamstrings, more severe pronation in one foot than in the other, and so forth. Incomplete healing of old injuries that you may have forgotten about also causes many asymmetries.

The best way to correct muscular asymmetries is by stretching and strengthening the muscles on either side of your body independently. If your left calf is tighter than your right calf, for example, simply stretch it more. And rather than perform standard squats, which can mask strength imbalances between the left and right legs and allow them to persist, perform lunges, which quickly reveal strength imbalances and allow you to correct them.

Skeletal imbalances such as asymmetrical arches and leg length discrepancies usually need to be diagnosed by a physical therapist. When discovered, such problems are generally managed through the use of special shoe orthotics.

Becoming a Runner

I believe that the single best way to become a better triathlete runner is to become a plain old runner for a short while and then return to triathlon. And the best way to do this is to train for and compete in a fall marathon. Running as frequently and as far as one does when training for a marathon is a wonderfully effective means of achieving the kind of skinniness I was talking about above. It will make you literally leaner, but it will also make you a more efficient runner and improve your running-specific endurance and aerobic capacity. While these changes will reverse themselves to a degree when you return to regular triathlon training, they will not reverse themselves entirely. I know this from experience. You will come back to triathlon from running as a better triathlon runner.

But why the fall? Of course, you can do a marathon anytime you like, however, autumn makes the most sense because focusing on running at this time will be least disruptive to your triathlon training and racing. Here's how to go about it. Do your last triathlon of the season in late July or early August (perhaps a little earlier than you would otherwise do). In the final several weeks of your triathlon training cycle, place a heavier emphasis on run training by performing an extra run workout each week and longer long runs. After completing your final peak triathlon, increase the frequency of your run training to six workouts per week. Perform as many swim and bike workouts in addition to these half-dozen runs as you care to do, but eliminate all cycling workouts in the final two weeks before your marathon.

Start doing two quality runs a week if you were not doing so already. Do a tempo or cruise interval workout (see workout descriptions below) each week. The other quality workout can be either speed repetitions or max oxygen intervals. Go for a long run every other week and increase its duration each time until four weeks before your marathon. Cover 20 to 24 miles in this peak long run. Do a final long run of 15 miles two weeks before race day. During the alternate weeks when you're not doing a long run, do a marathon-pace workout instead. Warm up, run for 60 to 90 minutes at your projected marathon race pace, and cool down. Taper for two weeks. Reduce your run training volume by about 40 percent two weeks before the race, and by another 40 percent in the final week of training. And there you have it.

Many triathletes, including some elites, have successfully practiced the strategy of becoming a runner in order to become a better triathlete. Olympian and three-time U.S. National Champion Hunter Kemper provides a good example. Kemper took up triathlon at age ten and won five consecutive IronKids National Championship titles on the strength of his formidable swimming and cycling abilities. With designs on turning professional one day, Kemper decided to forgo triathlon competition during his college years at Wake Forest University and focus entirely on running. It worked. By the time he graduated he was a 30-minute 10K runner, and as a pro triathlete, running was his greatest strength.

Run Workouts

As with swimming and cycling, the key to performing appropriate run workouts is mastering intensity. You can calibrate running intensity in almost exactly the same way I encouraged you to calibrate cycling intensity in Chapter 4. That is to say, the best place to start is by simply doing appropriately structured threshold and max oxygen workouts. A good threshold running workout is to run 18 to 24 minutes at a pace you feel you could maintain for 60 minutes and no more in race conditions. Make sure to warm up thoroughly before this and to cool down thoroughly afterward. A good max oxygen workout is four to eight intervals lasting four to five minutes each and run at a pace you feel you could maintain for no more than about 15 minutes in race conditions. Jog at recovery intensity for four to five minutes between intervals, and again, be sure to warm up and cool down.

Because threshold and max oxygen intensity represent very precise physiological circumstances, it's easy to *feel* —or at least to learn to feel—when you are indeed running at either of these intensities. In a word, threshold pace feels comfortable, but just barely. You should perform threshold workouts at the fastest pace that feels more or less comfortable the whole way through. You should feel moderately fatigued toward the end of the session, but little or no lactic acid burn.

Similarly, you should perform your max oxygen workouts at a pace that corresponds to your maximum capacity for controlled breathing. If you reach this state less than about a minute into each interval, you're going too fast. If you feel you could inhale and exhale a little harder without hyperventilating, you're going too easy. Also, if you perform your max oxygen workouts correctly, your last interval should be performed at the same pace as your first, and you should be sure that you could complete at most one more interval at the same pace.

You can enhance your mastery of run training intensity by using the objective measurement of pace and heart rate. Simply do your workouts on a 400-meter track and/or wearing a heart rate monitor, and pay attention as you train. Training on a track and monitoring your pace is particularly helpful because the controlled environment helps you maintain consistent efforts and makes measuring your progress easy, and also because it helps you project how fast you'll be able to run in upcoming triathlons.

As for the three remaining intensity levels, endurance intensity is anything below threshold level and above recovery level. However, most of your endurance training should be performed near the middle of it, well above recovery intensity and well below threshold intensity. Recovery intensity should just feel very easy while still being intense enough to qualify as exercise. Your speed pace need not be precise either. A good speed workout might consist of six to 12 intervals (depending on your fitness level) lasting 90 seconds each and separated by three or four minutes of recovery jogging. Your pacing is appropriate if you complete the last interval at the same pace as your first and you feel you could perform no more than one additional interval at the same pace.

If you have some experience as a runner, you may be accustomed to calibrating your pace for various intensity levels of training using recent race performances. This works quite well. Your threshold training pace should be 10 to 20 seconds per mile slower than your 10K pace—closer to 10 seconds per mile if you're a faster runner and closer to 20 seconds per mile if you're a slower runner. Your max oxygen pace should be zero to four seconds per 400 meters slower than your 5K race pace. And finally, your speed pace should roughly match your one-mile race pace.

Table 5.1 presents suggested run training paces for the three general categories of quality run workouts, based on 10K performance. Note the one-minute gaps between 10K times in the first column and understand that the difference between, say, a 39:30 10K and either a 40:00 or a 39:00 is not insubstantial. In other words, the suggested training paces offered here are only approximate.

However, since your appropriate training paces will tend to become faster as you improve and gain fitness anyway, you will always find yourself needing to evaluate your target pace for workouts against the subjective experience of completing these workouts. Over time you will develop a refined ability to micro-adjust intensity from one workout to the next and even within workouts.

Suggested Quality Run Training Paces

10K Run Time	Threshold Pace	Max Oxygen Pace	Speed Pace
(Minutes)	(Per Mile)	(Per 400 meters)	(Per 400 meters)
32	5:20	1:14	1:08
33	5:32	1:16	1:10
34	5:41	1:18	1:12
35	5:51	1:20	1:14
36	6:00	1:22	1:16
37	6:09	1:25	1:19
38	6:20	1:27	1:21
39	6:29	1:29	1:23
40	6:38	1:31	1:25
41	6:47	1:32	1:26
42	6:55	1:35	1:29
43	7:04	1:37	1:31
44	7:13	1:39	1:34
45	7:22	1:41	1:36
46	7:33	1:44	1:38
47	7:42	1:46	1:40
48	7:52	1:48	1:42
49	8:02	1:50	1:44
50	8:12	1:52	1:46
51	8:22	1:54	1:48
52	8:31	1:56	1:50
53	8:40	1:58	1:52
54	8:49	2:00	1:54
55	8:58	2:02	1:56
56	9:07	2:05	1:59
57	9:17	2:07	2:01
58	9:26	2:09	2:03
59	9:36	2:12	2:05
60	9:46	2:14	2:07

Table 5.1

Let's now take a look at several specific types of run workout—in fact, *every* type of run workout you'll ever need to do. The appropriate phases for each workout type are indicated between parentheses.

RECOVERY RUN

(BUILD, PEAK)

A recovery run is a very low-intensity run lasting between 20 and 45 minutes, but no longer. Whenever convenient, it should be performed on grass or packed dirt. The purpose of recovery runs is to accelerate the body's recovery from recent hard workouts by increasing blood flow. They're also good as taper workouts in the final days before a race, when you want to exercise lightly. For triathletes who are just starting, or who are starting over, there are no recovery runs, because even low-intensity workouts will stress the body. Highly fit triathletes can perform longer recovery runs of moderate intensity that serve the twin purposes of aerobic maintenance and recovery. However, due to the high-impact nature of running, both swimming and cycling lend themselves to recovery workouts much better than running does. So, in general, when you need a recovery workout, try to swim or bike rather than run.

ENDURANCE RUN

(BASE, BUILD, PEAK)

An endurance run is just your standard steady-pace run of moderate aerobic intensity, or "junk mileage" as runners often call it. But endurance runs are anything but junk. They are the very foundation of running fitness. You can't do any of the long runs or high-intensity workouts that maximize running fitness without having first performed a great many endurance runs and thereby established solid aerobic capacity and raw endurance. Endurance runs generally range between 20 minutes (for beginners) and an hour in duration. Any endurance run lasting much longer than an hour should be classified as a long run. Again, try to perform a set of strides, accelerations, hill bounding, or some combination of these drills following endurance runs once or twice a week throughout the year, except perhaps during the portion of the training cycle when you're doing speed repetitions.

LONG RUN

(BASE, BUILD, PEAK)

The long run is one of the most important workouts for runners and triathletes alike, and it is especially important for triathletes who compete in long-distance events. The primary objective of the long run is to increase your body's ability to burn fat and conserve carbohydrate fuel. Long runs should be performed at the same intensity as endurance runs and should last between 70 minutes and two and a half hours, depending on your training history, present fitness level, and the length of the longest peak triathlon in your present training cycle. Go for one long run each week or every other week throughout most of the training cycle, beginning in the middle of the base phase.

Always remember to carry a sports drink with you on long runs. Transporting more than about 16 ounces of fluid while running is not practical. This amount is adequate for 60 to 80 minutes of running, so when you run further, plan a refueling stop.

FARTLEK

(BASE)

A *fartlek* run is an endurance run in which you intentionally play with pace. (One of those supposedly little-known facts that everyone knows is that *fartlek* is Swedish for "speed play.") Simply begin running at a moderate aerobic pace, and when the spirit hits you, pick up the pace and maintain it until you feel like easing up again. The higher intensity efforts need not all be equal in intensity, but there should be some degree of method to the madness. I myself like to do 30- to 40-second bursts at speed pace and two- to three-minute efforts at threshold pace, with at least three minutes between any two pickups. The total run should last between 40 and 70 minutes. Fartlek runs are great workouts for the latter portion of the base phase when you're beginning to feel fit but it's not yet time for formal high-intensity workouts.

TEMPO RUN

(BUILD, PEAK)

Warm up with at least ten minutes of easy running at recovery pace. Run 16 to 24 minutes at threshold pace on relatively flat terrain with good footing and in good weather conditions. If you enjoy running on the track, you can do this workout there. Be very careful not to exceed your appropriate threshold pace. Cool down with at least 10 minutes of easy running. Do shorter tempo runs earlier in the training cycle and gradually increase their duration.

CRUISE INTERVALS

(BUILD, PEAK)

Cruise interval workouts are similar to tempo runs, but instead of containing one longer threshold effort, they contain a few shorter ones—for example, 2 x 12–20 minutes or 3 x 6–12 minutes. Breaking up your threshold work in this manner gives you a little more flexibility, because it's a little easier to do 2 x 10 minutes of threshold-pace running than 20 minutes straight. You can do shorter cruise interval workouts earlier in the training cycle, before you're ready for longer tempo runs, and do longer cruise interval workouts later in the training cycle, when you're in good shape and are able to handle more than 24 minutes of threshold-pace running in a single training session. Active recoveries between cruise intervals should last two to six minutes. Don't forget to warm up and cool down!

MAX OXYGEN INTERVALS

(BUILD)

After completing a thorough warm-up, do several max-oxygen-pace runs of appropriate duration separated by three- to four-minute active recoveries. Intervals should last between four and five minutes, which comes to 1,000 to 1,400 meters for most runners. I find it best to perform max oxygen intervals on the track, for the controlled environment. Less fit triathletes should do no more than four such intervals in any single workout. Highly fit triathletes can do as many as eight. To cool down, repeat your warm-up. Max oxygen interval workouts are extremely taxing, but they work wonders to increase both aerobic capacity and confidence.

SPEED REPETITIONS

(BUILD)

Speed repetitions represent the fastest running you will do as a triathlete. Their main purpose is to improve running economy, anaerobic metabolism, and lactic acid tolerance. Also, because they are much faster than race pace, they provide a psychological benefit by making race pace seem slow. Like max oxygen intervals, speed repetitions are most effective when performed on a running track. Individual repetitions should last between 30 seconds and three minutes, and so a typical set of speed repetitions includes high-intensity efforts ranging from 200 meters to 800 meters, with 400-meter repetitions being most common. The classic speed repetitions workout is simply 8–12 x 400 meters with three- to four-minute active recoveries. You can mix together repetitions of various distances or keep them all the same, as in this example. Avoid doing more than about three total miles of speed-pace running within any single workout.

HILL REPETITIONS

(BUILD)

Hill repetitions are speed repetitions with a twist—or a hill, rather. You can do them on a straight stretch of road or trail with a consistent, moderate grade, or on a treadmill set at an appropriate grade (6 to 8 percent). The advantage of doing hill repetitions on a treadmill is that you don't have to keep running downhill to start the next repetition, which can be hard on the knees and quadriceps. The ideal duration of each repetition is about 90 seconds. Do between four and ten of them, depending on your overall training volume. Warm up and cool down with at least ten minutes of recovery-pace jogging.

ROAD RACE

(BASE)

Participating in formal road running races (5K, 10K, and others) can serve two purposes. First, as I mentioned above, it can provide precise information about your current running fitness level, which you can then use to determine appropriate training intensities. Also, races are terrific workouts. They are very stressful on the body and take time to recover from, but precisely because they're harder than any workout, they can take your running fitness to the next level.

Always make sure to surround any running races you choose to do with a couple of easy days on either side, and avoid doing such races altogether when your training workload is already heavy enough.

BRICK WORKOUT

(BASE, BUILD, PEAK)

As I mentioned in the previous chapter, a brick workout comprises a bike ride followed immediately by a run, and it's a type of workout that is unique to triathlon and duathlon. There are many ways to approach a brick. Once more, I recommend doing one brick each week throughout most of the training cycle and varying the approach based on your location within the cycle. For example, during the early base phase you might do a moderately long ride followed by a moderately long run, both at endurance intensity. In the early peak phase, you might do a threshold ride followed by a tempo run. Feel free to mix it up, so long as the intensity of the two segments makes sense in terms of your present training needs and you make sure to count a high-intensity brick against the total number of high-intensity workouts you can handle in one week.

Recommended Run Training Parameters

This table suggests basic run training parameters for triathletes in each of four very general categories. Note that these categories do not distinguish among triathletes with different levels of ambition with respect to the type of event they're training for. A triathlete hoping just to finish a middle-distance triathlon, for example, need not train as heavily as one who's training for a breakthrough performance in a race of the same distance.

Category		Base Phase	Build Phase	Peak Phase
Beginner	Key Workouts	Walk/Run	Endurance Run	Brick Workout
	Weekly Mileage	6–10	8–15	10–18
Sprint	Key Workouts	Endurance Run	Max Oxygen, Speed Reps, Brick Workout	Tempo/Cruise, Brick Workout
	Weekly Mileage	12–25	16–25	16–25
Middle	Key Workouts	Endurance Run	Max Oxygen, Brick Workout, Speed Reps	Tempo/Cruise, Long Run, Brick Workout
	Weekly Mileage	16–40	20–40	20–40
Long	Key Workouts	Endurance Run, Brick Workout	Tempo/Cruise, Brick Workout, Max Oxygen	Long Run, Brick Workout
	Weekly Mileage	20–45	35–45	35–55

Table 5.2

Periodization of Run Training

Following is a concise characterization of the best way to approach your run training in each of the three main phases of the training cycle. In Chapter 6 I'll talk about how to mix together swim, bike, and run training in all three phases.

Base

Base phase running can be thought of as "training to train." In this phase, you seek to gradually increase your body's capacity for aerobic energy metabolism and for carbohydrate fuel conservation, which is the essence of endurance. You seek also to gradually increase the resilience of the bones, tissues, and joints of the lower extremities so that they do not develop overuse injuries now or later.

Your first running workouts in the base phase should be moderate in duration and fairly low in intensity. Gradually increase running volume while holding the intensity at a low level. Begin doing a weekly or biweekly long run and a weekly brick workout around the middle of the phase. At this time you may also begin to visit the upper region of the endurance intensity zones during the latter portion of your long run and when encountering hills during endurance runs. Perform a set of strides, accelerations, and/or hill bounding at the end of two of your weekly runs throughout the base phase. These will keep you sharp and will help to improve your form.

The end of the base phase is a good time to do one or two road races in order to ascertain your running fitness and determine appropriate paces for the initial quality workouts coming in the build phase. Besides these optional races and your strides, the only running you should perform at or above threshold intensity should occur in the context of occasional fartlek runs done toward the end of this phase.

Due to the high-impact nature of running, you need to be extra careful as you increase your run training volume during the base phase. Increase your weekly running volume by no more than 10 percent in any given week, and remember to practice step cycles, in which you increase the workload for two or three weeks and then cut back for one week to absorb the training you've just done. Increase your long run duration by no more than 10 percent every other week.

Build

In the build phase, you want to maximize your running workload by maintaining the training volume you built up to in the base phase and introducing a goodly amount of high-intensity training into your schedule. As you transition from the base phase to the build phase, quality workouts such as hill repetitions and max oxygen intervals should become your key workouts.

Perform just one quality run workout each week unless you're competitive and have done some heavy training in the past, and even if you fit this description, begin each build phase with just a single weekly quality run. One approach is to begin with a weekly speed-intensity workout such as hill or speed repetitions and, after doing a few of these, switch over to max oxygen intervals, which are more taxing and more triathlon-specific in their training effect. However, as I said in relation to cycling, you can reverse the order if you wish, or alternate the two types, and still make similar gains in fitness. If you do two weekly quality runs, do a speed-pace workout and a max-oxygen-pace workout. Another option, which is most appropriate for long-distance specialists, is to eschew speed-intensity workouts entirely and get what little speed-intensity training you need in the form of strides and fartlek. In this case, threshold-intensity workouts such as tempo runs and cruise intervals can take the place of speed-intensity workouts.

Again, your overall training volume should remain fairly consistent throughout this phase, but do practice step cycles. Maintain the duration of your long runs as well. Continue performing a weekly brick workout. You may also begin doing lower-priority races during this phase.

Peak

Your main objective in the peak phase is to maximize race readiness by emphasizing race-specific workouts and getting adequate rest, especially toward the end of the phase. Perform one threshold-intensity run per week throughout this phase, as this intensity level is close to race intensity for many triathletes in many races. In addition to these workouts, do a run at precisely your projected race pace (for the longest triathlon you have ahead of you) about once every other week.

If your final peak race is a long-distance event, or an event that will be challenging just to finish, your training volume and the duration of your long runs should begin once again to steadily increase in this phase. Otherwise, they should be held steady. Continue doing that weekly brick workout. Also, in this phase be sure to do at least a couple of triathlons prior to the peak triathlon that will conclude the present training cycle. These races will both reward and increase your fitness.

Within a week to three weeks of your final peak triathlon, perform a one- to three-week taper (the longer the triathlon, the longer the taper). Cut out the long runs and reduce total run training volume incrementally. Maintain the intensity of your quality workouts, but reduce the volume here as well.

Triathlon Slang

Like any subculture, triathlon has its own jargon. Actually, like the sport itself, triathlon jargon is mostly an amalgam of slang terms from the sports of swimming, cycling, and running. The ability to use this jargon appropriately and unselfconsciously is a symbol of belonging in the triathlon fraternity. Not understanding individual slang terms when they're spoken can make you feel like an outsider. Following is a list of common triathlon colloquialisms that you should add to your working vocabulary, supposing they're not there already.

Bag (v) To blow off a planned workout or race. Example: "I just couldn't get motivated, so I decided to bag it."

Banana hammock (n) An off-color term for bikini swimsuits for men. Example: "Make sure you wash my banana hammock before you return it."

Blow up (v) To reach a state of total exhaustion and sharply reduced ability to perform. Example: "I blew up at mile three."

Bonk (v) To reach a state of total exhaustion and sharply reduced ability to perform. Example: "Go on ahead. I'm bonking."

Bottom feeder (n) An unkind way of referring to a poor swimmer. Example: "I never swim there anymore—too many bottom feeders."

Crime fighters (n) A humorous term for bikini swimsuits. Example: "Check out my new crime fighters."

DNF (acronym) Stands for "did not finish." These letters appear next to the names of all nonfinishers in official race results, for all to see. The acronym is also used as a noun and verb. Example: "I DNF'ed. I don't want to talk about it."

Dolphin (v) A technique whereby a triathlete runs from the beach into the surf and dives forward, then stands, runs, and dives again, and so on, until he or she is out far enough to keep swimming.

Drop (v) To suddenly leave behind another cyclist on a training ride or in a race. Example: "I dropped her like a bad habit."

Flailer (n) Another unkind way of referring to a poor swimmer. Example: "I can't believe he swims in the 1:20 lane now. He used to be a flailer."

Fred (n) A cycling-specific term of derision synonymous with "loser." Example: "I don't want to ride with him. He's a total Fred."

Fresh (adj.) A state of feeling relatively nonfatigued. "I felt surprisingly fresh coming into T2."

Froggy (adj.) A state of feeling springy in the legs and well prepared for a hard workout or race. Example: "Look out, I'm feeling froggy today."

Grape hangers (n) Yet another off-color term for bikini swimsuits for men. Example: "Nice grape hangers, dude."

Hammer (v) To ride one's bike very fast. Example: "That chick hammers!"

Hit the wall (v) To reach a state of total exhaustion and sharply reduced ability to perform. Example: "I hit the wall on that last hill."

LSD (acronym) A running terms that stands for "long, slow distance." Note: The coincidental fact that a certain hallucinogenic drug shares the same acronym has been observed to death and should be left alone by everyone forevermore.

Mash (v) To struggle with too high a gear selection. Example: "Hey dude, shift down, you're mashing."

Newbie (n) A beginner. Example: "Take it easy on him—he's a newbie."

Noodle (v) To ride slowly and aimlessly. Example: "I feel like noodling today."

Off the front (adj) A state of being ahead of the main cycling pack, either on a training ride or in a race. Opposite: off the back.

Pack fodder (n) A poor cyclist. Example: "Pack fodder ahead."

Road rash (n) A bloody scrape or large scab resulting from a bike wreck.

Stud (n) A gender-neutral term for a talented triathlete. Example: "Karen is a stud runner."

Suck wheel (v) A negative euphemism for drafting. Example: "I'd be fresh still too if I'd sucked wheel the whole ride."

T1, T2 (abbreviation) Abbreviations for the first and second transitions in a triathlon. Also known as "swim-bike transition" and "bike-run transition." Example: "Matt Fitzgerald left T1 with a clear lead."

Tri-geek (n) Originally a term of disparagement used by single-sport swimmers, cyclists, and runners; now just a general synonym for "triathlete." Example: "The Saturday group ride I do has a pretty even mixture of roadies and tri-geeks."

Work (v) To cause a fellow or rival athlete to suffer during a training session or race. Example: "I worked him on the big hill."

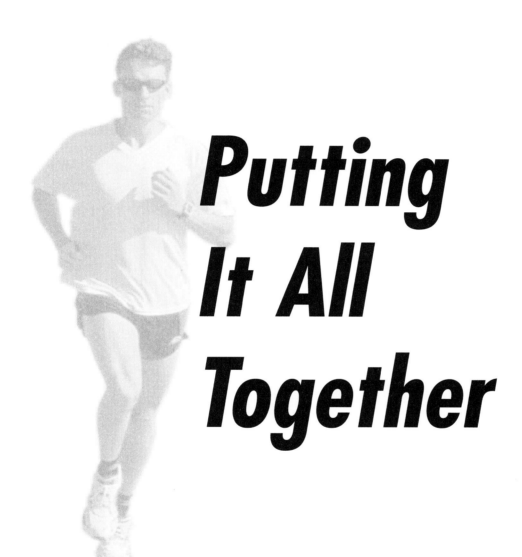

CHAPTER 6

Putting It All Together

Beginners can (and often do) get away with a spontaneous approach to training. When your general fitness and sport-specific adaptation levels are low, almost any kind of training you do will improve your conditioning and performance. But the fitter and more experienced you become, the more difficult it gets to find ways to improve still further. This is when planning becomes essential. *Lasting* improvement in triathlon requires a certain amount of knowing what you're going to do before you do it, and why. In this respect, triathlon is not unlike any other discipline, be it entrepreneurship or checkers. You need a strategy that looks a few steps ahead.

Unless you wish to hire a coach, you will need and want to make decisions and choices when it comes to planning your training. In other words, you will need to have the ability to design your own training program. This requires a little time and effort, but no more expertise than is represented in the eight general rules of triathlon training I shared in Chapter 1 and the more specific guidelines and recommendations offered in the present chapter.

When and How Much to Plan

Training plans can be quantified in terms of how far ahead they look and how much detail they include. The most immediate steps in any plan should include the greatest amount of detail, the most distant steps, the least. If you're training toward a specific peak race, you should know almost exactly what you're going to do next week in terms of training: number, order, duration, and types of workouts, and even approximate pace and split times. But when looking, say, 18 weeks ahead, you'll probably want to go no further than specifying a target workload and plotting your key workouts in the three disciplines, because you just can't know exactly what your body will want and need at that time. This is not to say that you'll necessarily always know this week what your body will want and need next week. On the contrary, if you're good at listening to your body, more often than not you'll find yourself tweaking many of your planned workouts immediately before and even while performing them, based on how you feel and what's going on. Nevertheless, it's still worth your while to plan specific workouts for the next week to four weeks of training, as there's a big difference between making adjustments as you go and making things up as you go!

I recommend scheduling no more (and ideally no less) than a full season (about eight months) of training at a time: no more than this amount because a single training cycle should last no longer than about 36 weeks, and you should not plan the next training cycle until you've had an opportunity to evaluate the present one; no less than this amount (ideally) because it will help ensure that your training has direction and is progressive. Plot your workouts in detail one to four weeks ahead. Beyond that, plan only the approximate volume of training and key workouts by type. It's okay to set goals that are more than a year out, as long as they're reasonable. For example, I decided that I wanted to do an Ironman triathlon three full years before I actually went out and did it. When establishing such long-term goals, however, just don't assume you can make a detailed plan for every step of the way from here to there. Nobody can see beyond the horizon.

The best time for planning, most triathletes find, is during the off-season (winter in most cases). The right time for planning of all forms is shortly before the new plan is scheduled to begin, and a training program designed to produce a summer peak should indeed begin in winter. In the case of triathlon, the brief transition period between the past season's final peak and one's return to base building after the holidays affords the most time and energy for reflection on the merits and flaws of the past season's training and for the establishment of goals and priorities for the coming season. Of course, it's perfectly feasible to plan and begin a training program at any time of year, as long as one obeys basic principles such as allowing oneself enough time to reach a fitness peak at the time of one's chosen peak race. But winter is generally the best time.

Beginner Triathlete's 12-Week Training Cycle for a Sprint Triathlon

Phase/Cycle/ Week	Mon	Tue	Wed	Thu	Fri	Sat	Sun
Base 1.1	Off	Swim E (0:20)	Bike E (0:30)	Walk/Run E (0:20)	Off	Swim E (0:20)	Bike E (0:30)
Base 1.2	Off	Swim E (0:20)	Walk/Run E (0:20)	Bike E (0:30)	Off	Swim E (0:20)	Walk/Run E (0:20)
Base 1.3	Off	Swim E (0:25)	Bike E (0:35)	Walk/Run E (0:20)	Swim E (0:25)	Bike E (0:40)	Walk/Run E (0:30)
Base 1.4	Off	Swim E (0:20)	Bike E (0:30)	Run E (0:20)	Swim E (0:20)	Bike E (0:30)	Walk/Run E (0:25)
Base 2.1	Off	Swim S (0:30)	Bike E (0:40)	Run E (0:20)	Swim E (0:30)	Bike L (1:00)	Run E (0:20)
Base 2.2	Off	Swim S (0:30)	Bike E (0:45)	Run E (0:25)	Swim E (0:30)	Bike L (1:00)	Run E (0:25)
Base 2.3	Off	Swim S (0:30)	Bike E (0:45)	Run E (0:25)	Swim L (0:40)	Brick (0:45/0:15)	Run E (0:20)
Base 2.4	Off	Swim S (0:30)	Bike E (0:40)	Run E (0:20)	Swim E (0:30)	Brick (0:45/0:15)	Run E (0:30)
Base 3.1	Off	Swim S (0:30)	Bike E (0:45)	Run E (0:30) Strides	Swim L (0:40)	Brick (0:55/0:20)	Run E (0:35)
Base 3.2	Off	Swim S (0:30)	Bike E (1:00)	Run E (0:30) Strides	Swim L (0:40)	Brick (1:00/0:20)	Run E (0:40)
Base 3.3	Off	Swim S (0:30)	Bike E (01:00)	Run E (0:30) Strides	Swim L (0:40)	Brick (1:00/0:20)	Run E (0:40)
Taper 1.1	Off	Swim S (0:30)	Bike E (0:45)	Run E (0:30) Strides	Swim E (0:30)	Off	Sprint Triathlon

S = Short Intervals, E = Endurance Workout, L = Long Endurance Workout

Table 6.1

Beginners cannot, of course, rely on past experience in planning their training, except inasmuch as they have participated in other endurance sports. Also, they seldom get the inspiration to train for a first triathlon in the dead of winter. Furthermore, few newbies are interested in spending many months preparing for their first triathlon experience, and with good reason: why devote that kind of time and energy to a sport you're not even sure you're going to like? For these reasons, most triathlon beginners choose (and are well advised) to train just eight to 12 weeks (depending on initial fitness) for a sprint-distance triathlon, and only begin thinking about long-term training plans afterward. Table 6.1 shows a sample 12-week buildup for a sprint-distance triathlon (500-meter swim, 15-mile bike, 3-mile run) that's appropriate for an inexperienced triathlete who is healthy and has a modest initial fitness level. A beginner who completes this training program and the goal race successfully should extend this basic training template through the remainder of the season and then construct a more extensive program for the next season.

Schedules and Journals

A training plan is not the systematic tool it should be unless it's recorded somewhere outside your head—specifically, on paper or a computer—in the form of a schedule. Likewise, the results of your past training will have only limited power to shape your future training unless they, too, are recorded on paper or a computer in the form of a journal. The memory is faulty.

A training schedule looks ahead, a training journal looks back, and so they meet in the present and are actually just two dimensions of a single tool. I suppose you could keep separate schedules and journals, but few triathletes do. It's more convenient to simply replace the information about what you've planned to do with information about what you've actually done, day by day, as you complete each workout. Most computer training software and applications work this way, and with paper it's as simple a matter as writing your schedule in pencil.

Table 6.1 provides an example of a typical training schedule format. As you can see, it looks a lot like an ordinary weekly planner, except that the chronology of the training plan is structured not by calendar dates but rather by phases, (step) cycles, and week numbers. For example, "Base 3.2" signifies the second week of the third step cycle in the base phase of training. Planning one's training in blocks of these kinds is a great way to give structure, organization, and direction to the plan, as well as to ensure that it adheres to the fundamental principles of training. I'll discuss how to plan phases and step cycles below. The most important piece of information in the schedule is the date and specific nature of the peak race. The rest of the information in the schedule is oriented toward this terminal point, and indeed the schedule itself would have no reason to exist at all if there were no designated peak race. On each day preceding that of the peak race, a workout is plotted by mode and type, or a day off is scheduled.

Table 6.2 shows a sample week in a typical training journal. It represents a week of build-phase training in a 36-week program created by a competitive triathlete with the usual time constraints who does mostly middle-distance races. The journal is kept in the very same planner as the 36-week training schedule. The athlete has simply substituted information regarding workouts planned with information about the workouts actually performed and added information about how the workouts felt as well as morning pulse. Recording information about mood, how the body feels during workouts, aches and pains, and so forth can help you evaluate your training retrospectively at later times. It does this by allowing you to link various training patterns with various effects. For example, you may find that you always begin to feel overtrained when your training volume exceeds a certain threshold, or when you use four-week step cycles rather than two- or three-week ones.

Measuring your morning pulse is a good way to track your health and fitness. As you gain fitness, your pulse will trend slowly downward, which is fun to witness. When you are tired, overtrained, or sick, your morning pulse will be higher than normal and you can adjust your training accordingly. Some triathletes—those who really dig planning —include additional information in their training journals, such as daily weight, weather conditions, and even food intake. Born planners are also inclined to schedule and log their training using fancy software designed for the purpose, which allows you to do neat stuff like download heart rate monitor data and make graphs that plot particular training variables against particular quantified effects. I've dabbled in these technologies and understand their appeal, but still prefer to take a simpler approach from day to day. The important thing is not exactly how you schedule and log your training, but *that* you do. It adds a dimension to the triathlon experience and has a direct, positive impact on your competitive results.

Sample Training Journal Page

Here's a sample week's training record for an experienced triathlete training for middle-distance triathlons.

Build 3.2	Morning	Evening
Monday **HR: 48**	Swim: 2,000 yards Main Set: 4 x 100 @ 1:30, 8 x 50 @ 0:43, 4 x 100 @ 1:35 (felt good, but shoulder still sore)	Stretching, strength training
Tuesday **HR: 47**	Stretching	Run: 7 miles easy (0:56) (a little tired from work)
Wednesday **HR: 48**	Swim: 2,200 yards Main Set: 3 x (200, 100, 50) 200s @ 3:20 100s @ 1:30 50s @ 0:43	Brick: 1:00/0:30 Bike: avg. 18.1 m.p.h. Run: 20 min. tempo, 10 easy
Thursday **HR: 48**	Stretching, strength training	Bike: 1:18 w/ Jimmy, 5 x 6:00 VO_2 intervals (hard but good)
Friday **HR: 47**	Run: 4 miles easy (31:30), 6 x 100m strides (pain in heel of right foot)	Bike: 1:00 hilly group ride (18.2 miles)
Saturday **HR: 49**	Open Water Swim: 1.8 miles @ 0:54 (shoulder better today)	Long Run: 12 miles @ 1:30 (legs a bit heavy, energy good)
Sunday **HR: 47**	Long Ride: 55 miles @ 3:10 (very strong, great week!)	Stretching

Table 6.2

Creating a Training Schedule

Five basic steps are involved in creating a training schedule: 1) choosing your peak races, 2) arranging training phases and step cycles, 3) determining volume and workload, 4) defining your key workouts, and 5) planning a typical week. Let's take a close look at each of these steps.

Step One: Choose Your Peak Races

As I've suggested, planning is oriented toward peak races. Consequently, as you begin the process of planning a training year, your first priority is to select one to three peak races, which are the triathlons where you wish to achieve the most challenging performance goals. Feel free to participate in many more triathlons and other endurance events, if you wish, but don't expect to achieve more than three peak performances within a single training cycle. It's just not done.

There's no definition of an appropriate choice for a peak race. You can choose to make any triathlon on earth your most important (or second or third most important) race for the coming season. But where many triathletes go wrong is in failing to actually peak for these events, or any others, because they have not oriented their training toward them. It is not enough simply to *hope* you're at your best for your most important races. There's little point in attaching any special value to these races unless you take measures to ensure you're ready to perform at the limit of your potential on the morning each race takes place. Your training cycle will not be a cycle at all, but rather a meandering, squiggly line, unless you hinge it on your peak races.

The chosen peak race that comes latest in the season should always mark the end of a training cycle. For this reason, it's helpful if your final peak race of the season falls in the later summer or early autumn. You can make this happen either by making your last race of the season a de facto peak race, or by choosing a late-season race over earlier alternatives as a final peak race. If you competed with a swim or cross-country running team back in school, you're familiar with the pattern of timing your fitness peak to coincide with the championship meets, which always occur at the end of the season.

The training cycle that ends with your final peak race does not have to be the only training cycle you plan and perform during the year, however. You can complete between one and three training cycles during a year, depending on how far apart your peak races fall and on personal preference. What I will call the classic approach is to perform just one, long cycle with a base phase that begins in early winter and ends in early spring, a build phase that picks up then and ends in early summer, and a peak phase that lasts from early summer until late summer or early autumn, at which time the final peak race takes place.

The only time it might be downright *necessary* to perform just one training cycle in a year is when you're training for a first long-distance triathlon and you're beginning at a fairly modest level of fitness. If any two peak races fall more than 12 weeks apart on the calendar, which is common enough, you have the option to complete two training cycles, one that ends with the earliest peak race and a shorter one that culminates with the final peak race of the season. You can just squeeze a complete, three-phase training cycle into 12 weeks.

Some triathletes like to plan some kind of winter peak, too, and this third peak is almost invariably in a sport other than triathlon, such as cross-country skiing or pool swimming. For goal-oriented athletes who can handle a lot of hard training, these off-season buildups represent an excellent way to maintain a high level of fitness year-round. Sooner or later, though, every athlete needs to chill out for a while. In fact, regardless of the number of peaks you plan for the year, you should plan an off-season gap between a pair of training cycles that lasts at least four weeks. I'll discuss what to do during these gaps in the final section of this chapter.

Step Two: Arrange Training Phases and Step Cycles

Once more, a complete training cycle contains three phases: base, build, and peak. The best way to arrange these phases in your training schedule is to work backward from the date of your final peak triathlon to today, or whenever you'd like your program to begin.

Each of the three phases can last between four and 12 weeks, depending on a variety of factors, including initial fitness, the amount of time available, and the length of the peak race it leads to (short, intermediate, or long). No phase should last more than 12 weeks, because your body can't continue to adaptively respond to the particular training stimuli that are emphasized in each phase for more than this amount of time. So, there's never any reason for a training cycle to last longer than 36 weeks, unless you're beginning at a very low level of fitness and wish to progress through a pre-base phase before entering the training cycle proper. But by the same token, in order to prepare for a truly optimal performance in an intermediate or long triathlon, you won't want your training cycle to include much less than a full 12 weeks of base, 12 weeks of build, and 12 weeks of peak training.

This is why I consider a 36-week cycle to be a standard triathlon training cycle. Thirty-six weeks are equivalent to about eight and a half months, or just the right amount of time to take you from a base beginning around New Year's to a final peak race in early September, which is perfect for most triathletes. In this approach, the remaining sixteen weeks of the year between Labor Day and New Year's would represent an off-season gap between cycles. This is about the longest gap you'd want to allow yourself, even if you work out consistently through most of it, as indeed you should.

You should do one long training cycle, lasting at least 24 weeks, once a year, no matter when your peak races fall, and this long cycle should always include a full, 12-week base phase. The base phase should always be equal to or greater in length than either of the other two phases, while the build and peak phases should be roughly equal in length. The long base is important because it is truly the foundation of the endurance athlete's fitness. It serves to transform all the hard work you did in the previous training cycle into a higher level of basic endurance fitness and prepares your body and mind for the high-intensity work that's coming in the build and peak phases. So, for example, if you plan a 25-week cycle, it might include a 12-week base, plus build and peak phases lasting seven and eight weeks (or visa versa), respectively.

Shorter cycles work best when they immediately follow a longer cycle. The most common use for shorter cycles is between peak races that fall within a single season but far enough apart within the season that a short break from high-intensity training between them is necessary. For example, suppose you wish to peak for an Olympic-distance triathlon in early June and for a half-Ironman triathlon in mid-September. In this case, you might wish to schedule a 32-week (long) cycle beginning in early November that prepares you for the first peak race, followed by a 13-week (short) cycle that picks up right after this race and leads to the second. This short cycle might comprise a five-week base phase, a four-week build phase, and a four-week peak phase that includes a one-week taper. Avoid planning any gaps between cycles during the racing season. Whether with one cycle or two, you should always be actively building toward a fitness peak until you've completed your final peak race of the season.

Once you've plotted the three phases in your training plan, you'll next want to work out the step cycles that fit inside them. As I suggested in Chapter 1, step cycles can last two, three, or four weeks, and their purpose is to establish recurring patterns of hard work and recovery that help you increase your fitness gradually and steadily over a long period of time. The length of your step cycles and the amount of volume variation they entail should depend on how your body responds and also on where you are in the training cycle. If you've never used step cycles before, I suggest you begin very conservatively. Start with either two-week cycles or three-week cycles and small weekly variations in volume. If the pattern you choose is or becomes unchallenging, move to a longer cycle or make the volume variations more substantial. When increasing volume from one week to the next, lengthen primarily your key workouts.

In the base phase, when you're doing minimal high-intensity work and trying to increase volume, go for longer step cycles and greater weekly volume increases (up to 10 percent). Cut back your volume by a modest amount (up to 10 percent as compared to the first week's volume) and start each new step cycle at a slightly higher volume level than you started the previous one. In the build phase, when your focus is on high-intensity workouts, it's a good idea to shorten the cycles and decrease the amount of volume variation from one week to the next (maybe 5 percent). By adding minutes mostly to your quality workouts (that is, by making your hardest workouts harder), you will find the overall workload increase from one week to the next quite noticeable. In the peak phase, keep the length of the step cycles the same, but hold the volume steady from one week to the next, except in the final week, when you should reduce volume by 5 to 10 percent. If you plan to race fairly frequently during the peak phase, reduce volume only during the weeks preceding races.

Your step cycles will not always fit neatly into your training phases. If the length of a given phase is not an even multiple of the length of your step cycles, you will need to make one step cycle a week longer or shorter than the others. Another factor that can disrupt the symmetry of your step cycles is races. Except for low-key races that you wish to train through, each of your other nonpeak races should be preceded by a recovery week so that you're well rested for it. But the chance that these races will always happen to fall at the end of a scheduled recovery week is slim. When they don't, you'll again have to make one step cycle longer or shorter than normal. For this reason, it's a good idea to schedule races far in advance whenever possible. Such adjustments will hardly ruin your training program if you make them sensibly. And keep in mind that when you do lengthen a cycle, the extra step does not have to be a step up in workload; it can be anything between a step up and a recovery week, depending on what you can handle at that time.

There are many ways to practice step cycles. Even among elite athletes there's quite a bit of variation in patterns practiced. But nearly all serious triathletes practice step cycles of some form or another. Don't be afraid to experiment with them. Start with a hunch and go from there. As long as you train hard enough during your hard weeks that you need an occasional recovery week, and you recover enough during these weeks that you're ready for even harder work during the ensuing week to three weeks, you're doing fine.

Step Three: Determine Volume and Workload

After establishing your training phases and cycles, you should next think about *how much* training you will perform through the course of your program. Three main factors will determine the volume of training that is appropriate: your training history, the amount of time you have available to train, and the length of your chosen peak events. Each of these factors influences training volume in its own way. Let's take a look at each.

Training History

As a general rule, the more endurance training you've done in your lifetime (without major hiatuses), and the more training you've done in the past several months, the more training you can handle in the next few months. The body cannot handle sudden and profound increases in training volume, either from week to week or from year to year. If you've trained 10 hours per week for the past four months, and next week you train 20 hours, you'll surely become sick, injured, or generally fatigued. Likewise, if you train 500 hours this year and then jump to 800 hours next year, even if you begin the new year at last year's average weekly volume level and only gradually increase it throughout the year, you will still probably become injured or generally fatigued.

From the time you begin to train for your first triathlon, you should gradually increase volume with each subsequent cycle until you reach a point where you don't wish to train more, or there's no practical way to do so. Of course, you can always *decrease* your training volume, as many triathletes do when returning to shorter triathlons after training for a long one. Plan your volume increases as a percentage of average weekly volume in your most recent cycle. For example, if you trained on average 10 hours per week in your most recent cycle, you may shoot for a 10 percent increase, or 11 hours per week, for your next training cycle. The triathletes who can safely increase their training the most (on a percentage basis, not in raw hours) are those who trained fairly lightly in their most recent cycle (less than 10 hours per week) but are still near peak form. If you fit this description, you can increase your average weekly volume by as much as 15 or 20 percent in your next cycle. If you trained very heavily in your last cycle (more than 16 or 17 hours a week), you should increase your average volume by no more than 5 percent, and only if you've remained near peak form. The more you've fallen off peak form since the culmination of your most recent training cycle, the less you should increase your volume for the next one.

If there's a golden rule of training volume, it's this: Be conservative. Now, to be conservative is not to lower your standards. The conservative approach is simply the most reliable way to reach a true fitness peak when you want it. One of the risks associated with planning your training as against doing it spontaneously is that it's much easier to plan too much training than it is to just go out and do too much. Be wary of this risk. By all means, train hard, and expect to experience moments during your training program when you feel worn out. But never let these moments last more than, well, a moment, before you rest and recharge.

For the most part, you should always feel you could do a little more throughout your program. Plan accordingly.

Time Available

Ah, yes: time available. This is a big issue for the great majority of triathletes. Very few triathletes with more than a year's experience are able to train as much as they'd like to, due to constraints on their time. This lament is different from the typical couch potato's excuse making. Triathletes who say they'd like to train more actually *would* train more if one or two of their other commitments vanished. Still, even triathletes with all the usual commitments (career, family, sleep) have enough time to train effectively for the sport, if not hard enough to win the Hawaii Ironman. Table 6.3 shows the minimum amount of time you should be able to commit to training in order to perform well in your peak races. How much more than the minimum you're able to do must depend on the specific nature of your daily commitments and how you handle the combined stress of these and your daily workouts. Be realistic. An extra hour of training per week will do you more harm than good if it becomes the straw that breaks the camel's back, where the camel is you and the broken back is something like chronic fatigue.

The best way to make up for limited training time is by being consistent. If you can work out nearly every day throughout the year, while getting enough rest and recovery, you may come out far ahead of your age-group competitors who train harder when they do train, but are inclined to miss a day here, a day there, and who slack off during the winter. Consistency can also mean less planned variation in volume, such that, while your maximum training volume is fairly low on account of your schedule constraints, you're never doing much less than the maximum. Elite triathletes without day jobs plan drastic volume variations into their programs. In an ideal world, so would you, but if you try to imitate such swings without increasing your maximum volume, you'll actually wind up undertrained. By holding volume more constant, you can close the gap between the elite's overall training volume and yours. Just be sure not to hold volume too constant, or your training will stagnate. Your training won't lead anywhere if it doesn't change. For this reason, if you fiddle with volume less, you may wish to fiddle with intensity more.

Remember that training volume is a function of the duration and frequency of individual workouts. You should vary the duration of workouts more than their frequency throughout most of the training cycle. Early in the base phase, when your fitness level may be relatively low and your primary objective is to gradually increase your training volume, you may wish to begin with a smaller number of weekly sessions and then add sessions one at a time until you reach the number of weekly workouts you want to maintain through the remainder of the training cycle (except perhaps during recovery weeks). From then on, changes in volume should result primarily from changes in the duration of individual workouts.

As for volume by discipline, in general, you should perform roughly equal numbers of workouts in each discipline each week. However, the bike workouts should be the longest, on average, and swims shortest, such that cycling accounts for 40 to 50 percent of your weekly training minutes, running 25 to 35 percent, and swimming 20 to 30 percent. The duration of each individual workout should be determined by your present fitness level, the length of the longest triathlon for which you're training and the nature of your goal for the race (finish, compete, or breakthrough), and the specific purpose of the workout. As a rule, if you train more than about 12 hours a week, your additional training hours should come primarily from doing longer long workouts and from greater workout frequency, and not so much from making *every* workout a little longer. Even for competitive long-distance triathletes, there's nothing to be gained from extending the average swim or run workout beyond 70 or 80 minutes or the average ride beyond two hours.

Length of Peak Races

Clearly, the longer your peak races are, the more training you'll need to do in order to prepare for a good performance. But even when race length is held constant, the more you train, the better you're likely to perform, up to a point. In other words, the volume of training you need to do just to make it through a long triathlon might be sufficient for a breakthrough performance in a middle-distance triathlon. For triathletes with limited time available for training, this is something to think about.

I refer you again to the table on recommended weekly training for triathlons of various distances. If you plan to compete at various distances, as most triathletes do, make sure your training is adequate for the longest of them. For this reason, it's wise to make the longest race of the training cycle the last race of the cycle (especially if it's a long-distance event). Also, when trying to determine whether you have enough time to train for a triathlon of a given distance, keep in mind that your peak week's volume will need to be 30 to 40 percent greater than your average weekly volume. It matters little that you have enough time for an average week of training for a given race if you don't have enough time for the hardest and most important weeks.

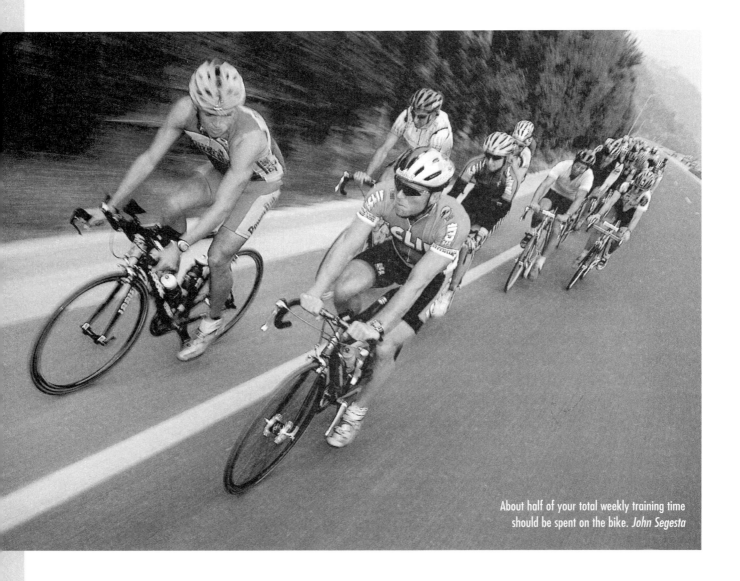

About half of your total weekly training time should be spent on the bike. *John Segesta*

Recommended Average Weekly Training Amounts for Various Peak Race Distances and Performance Objectives

Distance	Fun	Competitive	Breakthrough
Sprint	6 hrs / 6 workouts	9 hrs / 9 workouts	12 hrs / 10 workouts
Intermediate	8 hours / 7 workouts	12 hours / 10 workouts	16 hours / 12 workouts
Long	12 hours / 9 workouts	16 hours / 12 workouts	20 hours / 15 workouts

Table 6.3

Step Four: Define Your Key Workouts

Perhaps the most creative part of building a training plan is defining the nature of the key workouts you will perform in each phase. This will determine the style of your training program. It's not an anything-goes situation—only a small selection of key workout types is appropriate for any given situation. But there are choices to be made. Here are the primary choices by phase.

Base

The most important workouts in the base phase are your longer endurance swims, rides, and runs. The duration of these workouts should gradually increase throughout the phase and peak at the end of it. Before you begin your training program, figure out how long you want your longest swims, rides, and runs to be. Decide also how often you wish to do these workouts. At the least, you should do one swim, ride, and run every other week that's longer than any swim, ride, or run you've done previously in the training cycle, and do shorter long workouts in the alternate weeks. At the most, perform overdistance workouts three times every four weeks in each discipline.

Bike-run bricks are also key workouts in the base phase. Choices to be made with respect to these are how often to do them and whether to emphasize the bike or the run, or to alternate. I recommend doing a brick at least every other week and as often as weekly. It's not a bad idea to emphasize your weaker discipline in early-season bricks and then alternate between bike-focus bricks and run-focus bricks through the rest of the training cycle. In swimming, technique and power work are key in the base phase. At the least, do a long drill set incorporating some power intervals with fins and paddles (but not simultaneously) twice a week. At the most, do this plus an entire main set involving fins and paddles once a week.

Build

In the build phase, above-threshold-intensity workouts (that is, max oxygen and speed workouts) are most important. Speed-intensity workouts are optional in cycling and running. If you don't do formal speed-intensity workouts, make sure to incorporate some speed training into other workouts in the form of jumps (cycling) and strides and accelerations (running). Do at least four max oxygen workouts in cycling and running, and no more than eight. If you choose to perform speed workouts, do at least four and no more than eight. Separate workouts of the same type (max oxygen rides, speed runs, etc.) by at least a week and by no more than two weeks. Do at least one and no more than two above-threshold-intensity workouts (max oxygen and/or speed) each week in cycling and in running. My preference is to do a speed run and a max oxygen ride one week, a max oxygen run and a speed ride the next week, and so forth. You also have the option to begin doing threshold-intensity workouts in this phase if you like and can handle a lot of intensity. In swimming, your main choice is how often to do very hard main sets— once, twice, or at most three times weekly.

Peak

In the peak phase, long workouts are again key workouts, especially if you're training for longer triathlons or for any triathlon that will be challenging just to finish. Your choices are the same as they were in the base phase: how long? and how often? Your hardest workouts of the week should be threshold-intensity swims, rides, and runs—one of each. In addition to these workouts, you have the option of performing time trial workouts or other workouts at race pace. Second-priority races also qualify as key workouts in this phase, and here your choice is how often to do them. As in the build phase, you need to decide as well how often to do hard main sets in swimming, whether once, twice, or thrice weekly. In any case, your most challenging main set of the week should emphasize threshold intensity.

Step Five: Plan a Typical Week

The smallest recurring cycle in a triathlete's training program is the weekly cycle. The fifth and final step you need to take in planning a training cycle is to work out the structure of a typical training week. While each specific week of training is unique, for the sake of convenience and consistency, most of them should follow the same, basic structure, because every successful triathlete does so and it seems to work. This is one instance when blind conformity will only help you.

Begin this process by deciding how many workouts you wish to perform on a weekly basis. Next, figure out when you have time to work out, and how much time you have to work out when you do. Most of us have the greatest freedom on weekends. The next best opportunities tend to fall before and/or after work hours. Many triathletes are also able to do regular lunch hour workouts and find them to their liking. Label each workout opportunity according to the day of the week and whether it's before noon or after noon (unless you plan to do more than two workouts a day some days, in which case you should include a noon workout category, too).

When you've completed this process, it's time to schedule recurring sessions by mode. Try to plan roughly equal numbers of swim, bike, and run sessions, including the bike and run segments of your brick workout. If the total number of workouts you plan to perform in a typical week is not a multiple of three, use your judgment to decide in which discipline(s) the extra workout(s) should be, or simply change it each week. Do your best to distribute the workouts by mode throughout the week so you're never working out in the same mode twice in a row. If you plan to do supplemental stretching and strength training on a regular basis, don't forget to schedule these activities as well.

The majority of triathletes with normal weekends like to do a long run on Saturday and a long ride on Sunday, or vice versa, as these workouts tend to last too long to squeeze into a workday. While you won't be doing long rides and long runs every weekend, it's simplest to reserve space for them throughout the training cycle so that you're always doing a run or a ride on these days (morning or afternoon), be it long or short. The brick tends to be a longer workout as well, making it a good candidate for weekend placement, but you can't very well do a long run, a long ride, and a separate brick in one weekend, so you may choose to combine them in one way or another. Alternatively, during those portions of the training cycle when you're doing quality training, you can keep your brick workouts shorter and raise their intensity level so that one or both segments serve as quality sessions for the week.

After you've worked out the structure of a typical week, you need to adapt it for each phase and intraphase step cycle. For the most part, this will entail merely specifying the duration and type of workout slotted for each workout space in your typical week, but it may also entail the following: cutting back the number of workouts in the early portion of the base phase, as well as in taper weeks, and perhaps also in certain recovery weeks; reducing the frequency of strength workouts after the base phase; and incorporating other such deviations from the typical week structure that seem appropriate. Refer to the chapters on swim, bike, and run training for workouts that are most appropriate for each phase. When engaging in this process, try to buffer hard workouts with easier workouts and rest periods on either side, as much as possible. If you're doing double sessions a few or more times per week, these buffers will be 24 or 36 hours at least as often as they're 48 hours. Count both long- and high-intensity workouts as hard workouts. Note also that recovery from hard swims generally happens faster than recovery from hard rides, which happens faster than recovery from hard runs.

Table 6.4 shows a typical week structure that is very general but could be readily specified to any specific part of the training cycle, mainly by specifying the nature of the designated hard workouts. For example, if it's a base-phase week, the designated hard workouts will probably be endurance-intensity workouts in cycling and running, and interval workouts emphasizing technique and/or power work in swimming, and none of these workouts should be all that hard, especially in the early portion of the phase. If it's a build-phase week, the hard swim might be mixed intervals, the hard ride a set of long hill intervals, and the hard run a set of max oxygen intervals. If it's a peak-phase week, the hard workouts might all emphasize threshold-intensity training.

This weekly format can also be specified to any individual triathlete, with a few modifications. The sample week presented has 10 workouts (three swims, three runs, three rides, and a brick), making it appropriate for triathletes training for a short-course breakthrough, intermediate-distance competitiveness, or a long-distance finish, depending on average workout duration. Those wishing to do fewer workouts could customize this template by pulling out one or more easy workouts and perhaps also by making one or more of the hard workouts easy. Those wishing to do more workouts would want to add one or more workouts; whether they're hard or easy is up to the individual.

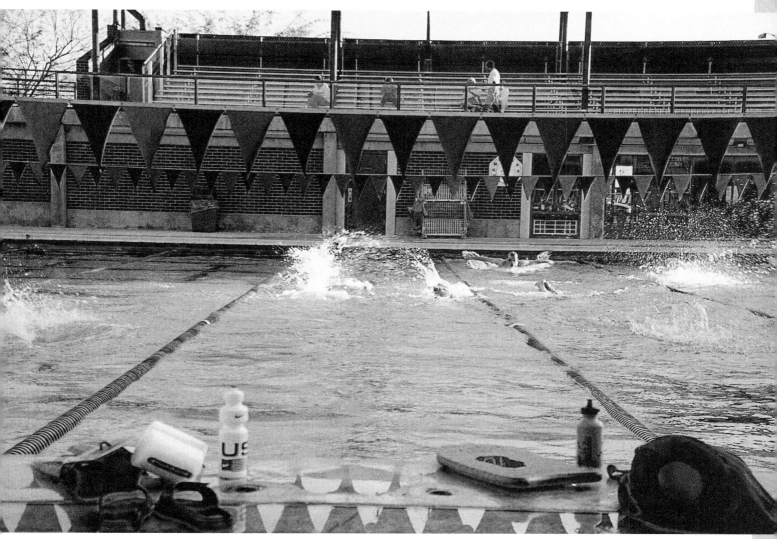

Group swim workouts are great, as long as their schedule and structure fit into your individual training plan. *John Segesta*

An Example of How to Structure a Typical Week							
	Mon	**Tue**	**Wed**	**Thu**	**Fri**	**Sat**	**Sun**
Morning	Easy Swim	Hard Run	Hard Swim		Easy Run	Long Swim	Long Ride
Afternoon		Easy Ride	Easy Run	Hard Ride		Long Brick (run emphasis)	
Table 6.4							

Making Adjustments

If you can make it through a 36-week training cycle without making any adjustments to your plan, call it a miracle. In other words, anticipate the need to make lots of little adjustments and perhaps one or two not-so-little adjustments as you progress through your training program, no matter how carefully planned. Minor adjustments will be required due to such things as travel, feeling better or worse than expected on certain days, distractions from other domains of your life, and a little caprice. Let the adjustments you choose to make in such circumstances be guided by common sense, an honest appraisal of your mind's and body's needs, and your knowledge of sound training principles and practices.

Major adjustments are required as a result of unplanned lapses in training caused by illness, injury, or protracted distractions from other domains of your life. The specific nature of the adjustments that such lapses require depends on many factors, including their length, when they fall in the training cycle, and the nature of the illness or injury. Generally, when you miss about a week of training and come back with a sound body, you'll find no significant adjustment necessary. If you miss a couple of weeks and come back sound, you'll probably want to give yourself another full week to return to form with slightly toned-down workouts. Longer lapses may require an adjustment in your race plans. At the very least, you will probably need to replan the remaining weeks of your program in such a way that the training carries you from your *current* level of fitness to the highest fitness peak you can manage in the time available. Don't make any decisions one way or the other, though, until after you've resumed seminormal training for a week or 10 days and assessed how much fitness you've lost.

What to Do Between Training Cycles

As I mentioned above, I recommend that you plan an intercycle gap lasting at least four weeks, and as many as 16 weeks, after your final peak race of the season. The main purpose of these gaps is to give your mind and body an earned rest. Their secondary purpose is to give you the chance to enjoy some alternative kinds of activity that you have little time for during the training cycles.

Whether your planned gap is short or long, you should start it by taking no less and little more than two weeks away from all forms of exercise. Go cold turkey. Taking fewer than 14 days off (completely off) will not result in the degree of mental and physical rejuvenation you need to stay strong and motivated for the next 50 weeks. Taking more than 14 days off will result in more than the ideal amount of detraining. Following this sedentary period, enter a period of informal, enjoyment-oriented exercise, preferably involving at least one activity other than swimming, road cycling, and running. Options include skiing, mountain biking, basketball, surfing, and strength training.

This period of playful exercise should then gradually phase into a period of pre-base training, unless you've planned a very short gap, in which case you'll phase right into base training. Actually, pre-base and base training are the same, except that in the former there is no real emphasis on building volume. During the pre-base period, do only low-intensity swim, bike, and run workouts that develop technique and strength rather than raw endurance. Continue to mix in other forms of endurance exercise such as snowshoeing if you wish. This is also the best time of year to develop a reserve of muscle strength through functional strength training. Do two or three such workouts per week during the pre-base period and the early portion of the base phase. I'll say more about how to incorporate functional strength training into your training program in Chapter 8.

The Lifelong Triathlete

A couple years after Mark Allen retired from triathlon, I bumped into him at a gym where we both had memberships. During our brief chat, I asked him what he was doing for exercise these days (besides lifting weights, which I could see for myself). "Surfing," he answered. I asked if that was all. He said, "More or less." He told me he hadn't run more than 45 minutes at a time since he quit racing.

While this news shocked me initially, after reflecting on it, I decided it made sense. For Mark, triathlon was all or nothing, because his all was so extreme as to have redefined our notion of the possible. He sacrificed everything to the quest for greater endurance for 14 years, and when he was done, he was done. There would be no casual dabbling in multi-sport. He would surf.

Mark Allen really needed to leave triathlon behind, but in this respect, as in so many others, he is an exceptional case. Unfortunately, though, all too many age group triathletes do the same thing. After first catching the triathlon bug, they train and race with increasing zeal for four or five years, and then they burn out completely, quit, and get soft (which is another key difference between the typical triathlon burnout and Mark Allen, who remains active and fit even without formal training).

High turnover is triathlon's dirty little secret. I'd like to see more triathletes remain triathletes for life, the way runners seem to do. In concept, this is easy: just keep swimming, cycling, and running, however casually, and showing up for the occasional race, if only just for the camaraderie. What stands in the way of this for so many triathletes is the kind of all-or-nothing attitude that, however appropriate for the likes of Mark Allen, is not helpful to folks like us. For a great many triathletes, the desire to improve becomes the primary motivator immediately after the desire to finish a triathlon has been satisfied. Improvement comes easily at first, but becomes increasingly difficult over time. You must train, focus, and sacrifice ever more. And even then, sooner or later, you reach a limit. The typical triathlete can improve gradually for many years, but not forever, and most amateur triathletes run out of time for improvement before they run out of ability.

For this reason, improvement can't be your only strong motivation to stay in the sport of triathlon, if indeed you're going to do it for the long haul. But what else is there? Well, the way I see it, improvement is just one form of discovery, and discovery should be every triathlete's primary motivator, because there's no limit to the amount of learning and growing you can do through the use of your body. And the joy of discovery is truly what motivates every new triathlete in the very beginning, before the desire to improve has a chance to emerge. Becoming faster is hardly the only way you can reach new places as a triathlete. Through awareness and accumulated experience, you can continually refine your training methods for decades, long after you've passed your so-called physical prime, and perhaps become a standout in the higher age groups even though you were middle-of-the-pack in the lower ones.

You can also continue to increase your triathlon-related knowledge base throughout your life by delving into exercise physiology, nutrition, bike technology, and so forth. You can keep trying new things by doing triathlons in different locations around the world and branching out into sports and activities like bicycle touring, cross-country skiing, and adventure racing. You can give back to the sport by mentoring or coaching other triathletes, as Mark Allen himself is now doing.

Don't become another triathlon burnout. Keep discovery as your primary motivator. You'll enjoy endless new experiences and personal growth, not to mention, you'll probably live as long as Noah!

CHAPTER 7

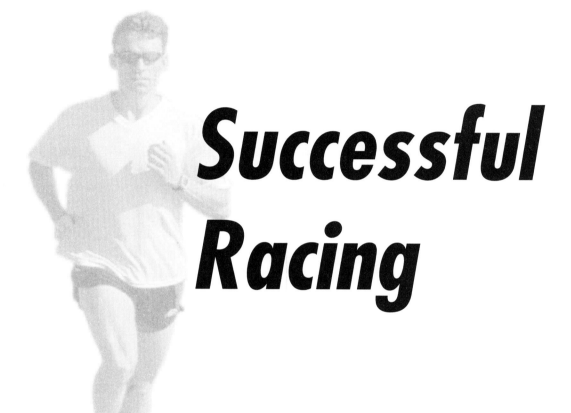

Successful
Racing

*T*he Chicago Triathlon is the largest triathlon in the world. As such, it has a larger transition area than any other triathlon. When it's staged each summer, nearly 5,000 bikes and other gear fill row after row of racks in a sprawling parking lot off Lakeshore Drive. In the 1996 staging of the race, a local age-grouper named Jim (last name withheld to protect his dignity) exited the water and jogged the long path into this homogenous maze feeling a little disoriented, but otherwise pretty good. He stopped running when he thought he'd gotten to the row containing his bike and peered along it, but did not see his own. So he jogged a little further, stopped at another row, and repeated this behavior. Again, he failed to recognize his bike among the many in the row. He then jogged back the way he'd come, looking worried. Once more, he paused at the head of a row of bikes, but this time, he chose to turn the corner and jog along the row, eyeing each transition spot individually, but it was not his row. His face now a mask of abject panic, Jim continued searching for his transition spot for a full five minutes—an eternity under such circumstances—before finally locating it. By then, literally hundreds of his competitors had passed him. Worse, this whole episode was recorded by a video camera, and a viewing of the tape of Jim's comical meltdown has become an annual Chicago Triathlon post-race party tradition.

What is the moral of this story? Well, perhaps there's more than one, but the moral I wish to highlight is this: All the preparation in the world means little if you fail to execute properly on race day. Had Jim rehearsed coming into the transition area and finding his bike before the race, he probably would not have lost several minutes and who knows how much energy circling it during the race, and he would have gone home happier (although, on the downside, the event's post-race party would have been deprived of a highly crowd-pleasing entertainment). Wasting five minutes looking for one's bike is just one of many kinds of mishap that can spoil one's triathlon, despite a high level of fitness. Rehearsing transitions is just one preparatory measure among many that have nothing to do with regular training but are critical to successful racing.

By no means is racing the whole point of pursuing the triathlon lifestyle, yet at the same time it's difficult to achieve the fullest satisfaction in the sport without the occasional positive racing experience, which we might define as a race performance that takes full advantage of good preparation. Beyond proper training, successful racing depends on your performing specific preparatory measures in the final weeks, days, and hours before the race, and on racing smart from start to finish.

When to Race

The best time to race is, naturally, at the end of the training cycle that you have presumably created to prepare yourself for a specific goal triathlon. You will never be more prepared to perform at your best than after completing a full training cycle and tapering period. For this reason, you should always try to arrange training cycles such that they terminate with your most important race, supposing you plan to do a few races in a cycle, and you should make your training most specific to this race, if you plan to do races of more than one length or type.

I probably don't need to say this, but I recommend that you consider one triathlon per season as a minimum racing requirement, because having a concrete goal before you will give meaning and direction to your training. If you wish to achieve the best possible performance in your peak race, you should do two or three other triathlons earlier in the training cycle as a part of your training. Competing in triathlons contributes to your triathlon fitness in a way that no mere workout can match, and every triathlon you do provides experience that you can apply in your next one. This is not to say that you can't pursue maximum performance in these nonpeak triathlons as well. You certainly can. But even if all you really care about is your peak race, doing two or three triathlons earlier in the training cycle is a good idea.

Triathletes can manage no more than two or three true *peak* performances each year. This limitation has both physical and psychological bases. A true fitness peak requires a lengthy period of physical preparation, lasts only a short time, and must be followed by a period of regeneration and rebuilding. That's the physical side of it. But breakthrough performances also require a state of mental preparation that also cannot be frequently achieved. First of all, it's difficult to be mentally ready for a peak performance without the confidence that comes from knowing you're physically ready. Also, triathletes (and all other athletes, for that matter) tend to perform best in those events that they've anticipated most and longest, and to which they consciously attach more importance than they do to other competitions. For these reasons, you should choose no more than three races each year in which you expect to perform at your very best.

Avoid racing when you don't have a good reason to race. There's no point in crossing the starting line unless you intend to give a full effort, and giving a full effort in triathlon is sufficiently taxing that it needs to be somehow worth all the suffering you experience during the race and the time you spend recovering afterward. You should have a clear sense of the purpose of your racing each time out. There are three distinct purposes you can assign to a triathlon. First, there are those triathlons in which you hope to achieve a peak-level performance; second, there are those triathlons in which you wish to perform your best, but which are not timed to coincide with a physical and mental peak; and third, there are those triathlons that you do for the sake of developing your race sharpness in anticipation of a coming peak race. These are all good reasons to compete. Making good on a bar bet ("Hey, I'll bet you can't stay out with us all night and then do that triathlon they're having at the lake tomorrow") is one example of a *bad* reason to compete.

Age group triathletes do not often over-race, but I'll warn you against it nonetheless. The definition of over-racing is not quantitative (as in, "doing x or more triathlons in y time span is over-racing) but qualitative: You're racing too much if you're not racing better each time. Over-racing leads to poor racing in either of two ways. On the one hand, racing too much can interfere with your training, as you need to rest before racing in order to perform well, and after racing in order to recover enough to return to hard training. If you race week after week, you won't be able to get in much quality training beyond what you get in the races themselves. As a result, before long your fitness will stagnate and your race performances will begin to suffer. Or, you could wind up in the same place by trying to maintain a normal training schedule despite frequent racing by limiting pre-race rest and post-race recovery. In this case you'll be fatigued for workouts and races alike.

This is not to say that you should never bunch together a few (shorter) triathlons in a relatively short span of time. In fact, during the peak phase of training, this can work out quite well, as your goal in this phase is to do highly race-specific training and otherwise rest. But avoid racing within three weeks of a peak triathlon. Also, as a general rule, avoid doing triathlons during the base phase of training and do no more than one or two (sprint- or intermediate-distance) triathlons a month during the build phase. And, of course, the longer your races are, the fewer total races you should do.

Many triathletes enjoy participating in occasional nontriathlon races such as 10K runs, mountain bike races, and open water swims. These races can provide excellent workouts, the motivation that comes from variety, and the opportunity to shine in your strongest discipline or gain strength in your weakest. Just be sure that each of these competitions serves a definite purpose, too (such as any of those I just named), and that it neither interferes with your normal training nor takes you beyond the overall workload you can safely handle. Just as you would do with training volume, always take a cautious approach toward increasing the amount of racing you do from one training cycle to the next, if indeed more racing is what you desire.

The Art of the Taper

As I've mentioned previously, the period of relative rest that precedes a race is called a taper. A well-executed taper increases your blood volume, maximizes carbohydrate fuel storage, increases aerobic enzymes, and enhances tissue repair, thereby rendering you better prepared for a peak performance. How long and how much you taper should depend on a few factors—namely, the volume of your preceding training, the length of the coming race, and the purpose of the race. The greater the volume of training you've been doing, the longer your tapering period should last. Also, the longer the coming race, the longer your taper should last. When the purpose of a coming race is sharpening for a later race, your taper can be shorter and less pronounced.

For short triathlons, your taper period can last four days to a week. For middle-distance triathlons, a week to two weeks of tapering is typical when a peak performance is sought. For long-distance triathlons, the taper can last two or three weeks. Reduce your training volume by 30 to 40 percent per week of tapering. For example, if you're tapering two weeks for a peak half-Iron triathlon and you did 20 hours of training in the last heavy week before the taper, you might do about 13 hours of training in the first week of tapering and about eight hours in the final seven days before the race.

Reduce your training volume primarily by performing shorter workouts and only secondarily by performing fewer workouts. You should cut back on your high-intensity training no more than you cut back on overall volume (about 30 to 40 percent each week). Although intuition might tell you to eliminate high-intensity training from your schedule when tapering, studies have shown that eliminating high-intensity training from one's schedule entirely in the period before a race results in lesser performances than doing a modest amount of high-intensity training during this period. However, don't perform any taxing quality workouts within three days of a race. In these last few days of tapering, limit your high-intensity work to several sprints in the pool and on the bike and several strides or accelerations on foot. If you're going to take a complete day off during race week, consider doing it two days out rather than one day, as some triathletes have a tendency to feel a little flat after a day of complete inactivity.

Many triathletes taper too little, not because they don't know any better, but because they just can't fully accept the idea that doing so little training will make them stronger. I've struggled with this form of paranoia myself. But the fact is, in most instances you'd race better after a week of no exercise than you would after a week of normal or only slightly reduced training. Tapering works.

Final Preparations

Besides tapering, there are several other preparatory measures you should take in the days preceding a triathlon. Most generally, you should get plenty of sleep and keep your stress level as low as possible. Of course, you should always get plenty of sleep and keep your stress level as low as possible, but when an important race is approaching, addressing these health needs is particularly important. When you fail to get sufficient sleep, your immune system is suppressed and your aerobic capacity is diminished. Needless to say, these consequences do not boost one's chances of achieving a breakthrough race performance. Stress, too, suppresses the immune system, and it can even cause injuries. Stress increases muscle tension in the body, which can lead to breakdown in tissues and joints that have been teetering on the edge of overuse. Because final preparations for a triathlon can themselves be a powerful stressor, triathletes frequently come up sick or lame within days of scheduled races. Take whatever measures you can to limit stress at such times, for example by taking a day off from work or asking your spouse to kindly handle one or two of your normal domestic responsibilities for a short time.

Like sleeping well and limiting stress, eating right is another habit that you should maintain at all times, but which becomes particularly important in the period before a triathlon. Your most vital specific nutritional needs in this period are maximum carbohydrate fuel storage and complete hydration. If the coming race will last less than two hours, continue eating your normal diet containing about 60 percent carbohydrate. For longer events, you should practice one of two carbohydrate loading protocols that endurance athletes frequently use, and which I will describe in Chapter 10. Drink about one ounce of water per kilogram (2.2 pounds) of body weight each day until the final day before your event, when you should drink an extra glass or two. Have drinking water accessible everywhere you go, or stay.

The taper period is also a good time to rehearse race transitions and swim starts and exits, especially if you're relatively inexperienced in triathlon racing. You can get a solid, race-specific swim workout by simulating the first and last 100 yards of the swim several times. Put on your wetsuit, if you'll be racing in one, and simply charge from the beach into the water, break through the surf (if there is a surf), and swim hard for roughly 100 yards. Then turn around, swim back to shore, and run onto the beach. To practice transitions, set up a makeshift transition spot just as you plan to set it up for the coming race. First practice your swim-bike transition several times. You can combine your swim exit practice with your swim-bike transition practice if you wish. Then practice your bike-run transition several times.

About one week before your race, give your bike a basic tune-up, or have a mechanic do so. It doesn't have to be a major overhaul. Just clean it thoroughly, lubricate the drive train, adjust bolts, and do such things as replace handlebar tape if necessary. Always race on new or almost-new tires. Install these a day or two before your race and ride on them once or twice to make sure there aren't any problems. Many triathletes like to make new equipment purchases they've been contemplating just in time to use them in a triathlon. This is fine, but again, test all new equipment purchases before giving them a real test in a competitive environment. For that matter, you should use the taper period to test any and all non-gear-related strategies and approaches you intend to try in an upcoming race as well. For example, if you wish to try taking glycerol before racing, as many endurance athletes do to increase water retention, then try taking glycerol before one or two longer morning workouts beforehand.

A great way to prepare mentally for a triathlon in the final weeks is mental rehearsal, or visualization. This entails finding some quiet time to sit or lie down, close your eyes, and imagine yourself swimming, cycling, and running with strength and confidence in the context of your upcoming race. Try to make these meditations as concrete and sensually detailed as possible—an effort that will be helped greatly if you have some familiarity with the course, but which is still feasible if you do not. While you want your mental rehearsal to be positive, don't make it unrealistically so. For example, rather than imagining that you feel no fatigue, even at the end of the race, imagine yourself fighting through fatigue and staying focused despite discomfort. Take yourself through the entire race, start to finish, in condensed form. Play some inspirational music if you like. (I like to choose a "theme song" for each important race I prepare for.) Do this at least several times, and as often as every night, right up until race eve.

Finally, I recommend that you get a few sports massages in the final weeks before any important race—perhaps one per week for three weeks. These will relieve tight spots in your muscles and thereby help keep you injury-free during this critical time, and may even enhance your performance on race day. Ideally, you'll be getting sports massages regularly, in which case you'll only want to avoid getting one too close to race day, as athletes commonly feel a little sluggish the day after a massage. Three days out is probably the perfect time for a final rubdown. If your massage therapist has been working on an injury, have him or her back off doing deep tissue work in this area at least two or three weeks before you race.

Traveling to Races

Traveling to races, especially by plane, can be a major hassle, but if you approach it systematically, this hassle can be minimized. Begin by gathering as much information as you can about the race, and reviewing it carefully. Take note of race packet pickup time and location, directions to this site and to the actual race site, if it's not the same, time and location of any pre-race athletes' meeting that might be taking place, hotels offering special rates to participants, and so forth. Even seemingly trivial details such as whether parking permits are offered or required for race site parking on race morning deserve your careful attention, or else they could become anything but trivial at the last moment. If you're not much of a planner and someone who's traveling with you is, ask this person to take charge and offer to make it up to him or her somehow.

Keep a checklist handy that you can refer to when packing for all of your races. See Figure 7.1 for a sample checklist. Give special attention to bike transport. If you're flying, investigate airlines' bike transport policies before booking an itinerary. (I have to say, most airlines are just plain prejudiced against cyclists—they charge $50 or more to transport a bike one way, while items that are just as large, such as some musical instruments, go free.) Purchase a high-quality bike case and pack it according to instructions (then tell the check-in attendant it's a tuba). For ground travel, the same principle applies. Use a high-quality trunk rack, roof rack, or a case that you can store inside your vehicle, and use it properly. Before departing, make the effort to locate a high-performance bike shop located near the race venue just in case something does happen during transport or some last-minute need materializes.

Triathlon Packing List

Swim Stuff	Run Stuff
Swimsuit	Training shoes
Triathlon suit	Racing flats
Goggles	Socks
Backup goggles	Running shorts
Swim cap	Running tops
Wetsuit	Hat/visor
Body lube	Fuel belt
	Race belt

Bike Stuff	Other
Bike	Towels
Shoes	Transition bag
Shorts	Energy bars, gels, drinks
Jerseys	Sandals
Helmet	Warm-up suit
Sunglasses	First-aid kit
Bottles/hydration	Sports watch
Spare tube	Lubricant
Tire pump	Body marker
Tools	USA Triathlon license
Aerobar	Emergency cash
Cyclometer	Heart rate monitor
Race wheels	Race information packet
	Sunscreen, lip balm

Table 7.1

Consider squeezing in a modest workout just before you leave. This will help prevent cabin fever during your journey and allow you to worry less about getting an opportunity to work out soon after your arrival, which is often difficult. (Triathletes have a funny way of viewing air travel as time travel, as though they could actually get out of shape flying from New York to California.) If you are flying, get up and walk around the cabin every 20 minutes or so to keep your blood circulating. If you're driving, make frequent pit stops. Take along plenty of water and healthy foods such as fruit and homemade sandwiches, as finding healthy food while traveling can be next to impossible. If you're crossing time zones, consider taking melatonin pills to minimize the effects of jet lag. Melatonin is a natural hormone that induces sleep and adjusts sleep cycles.

Plan to arrive in the race city or area early enough that you can do everything you need to do there prior to the race without rushing, yet not so early that you start needing to fill time with something—anything—other than endless thoughts about the upcoming race! For a typical Sunday morning triathlon, a Friday afternoon arrival is about right. Exceptions are cases when you wish to do some pre-race tourism or when you need to acclimatize to heat or considerable altitude change. When traveling from a cool or warm climate to a very hot (and possibly humid) climate to race, be aware that full acclimatization takes 10 to 12 days. Your performance will definitely suffer if you don't allow yourself this opportunity. Do only light workouts during the first three or four days (or do only light workouts outdoors and do the rest of your training indoors) and increase your fluid intake. You can always adapt ahead of time by working out in heavy clothing or in a warm indoor environment for several days before you travel to a hot race venue. It sounds odd, yet endurance athletes have used this strategy with great success for decades. Proceed cautiously if you do try it, however, as this practice brings with it the same risks of dehydration and heat stress as training in high atmospheric temperatures does. Like heat adaptation, adapting from a low-altitude environment (under 2,000 feet) to a high-altitude race location (above 5,000 feet) and vice versa requires at least 10 days.

If you should choose to spend several days in the race area before racing, make sure to plan for workout opportunities, for example by selecting a hotel that has an arrangement with a nearby health club with a pool and indoor cycling. An alternative to staying in hotels that many triathletes enjoy taking advantage of is home stay, which entails boarding at the home of a stranger who for whatever reason has volunteered to assist the race director in this way. Some race directors actively encourage members of their community to open their homes to visiting triathletes. There is no charge involved. Usually, those who participate will bend over backward to be helpful to you and expect nothing in return except the opportunity to get to know you a little bit. Contact your race directors to find out whether home stay is an option for the out-of-town triathlons on your schedule. Another option is to contact any triathlon clubs that may exist in the race area and ask whether its officials or members offer home stay.

Consider staying in a hotel the night before a race even if the triathlon is being held in your area. One reason to do this is to get *really* close to the race start, and thereby get a little extra sleep. Another reason is to avoid distractions and stimuli in your home environment that might keep you awake. I was once kept awake until 2:00 A.M. on the night before a race by a beer party at my neighbors' place.

The Final 24 Hours

A few years ago, I flew to New Orleans to cover and compete in the U.S. Duathlon National Championship. I had never been to the Big Easy and, well, I couldn't help myself. I stayed out all night in the French Quarter and the next morning lined up at the race start having had a 20-minute catnap and no breakfast of any kind, unless you count last call.[*] Needless to say, I suffered.

I share this story to illustrate the point that there is a great deal you can do to screw up a race in the final 24 hours before it happens, not all of it so blatant as getting drunk and refusing to sleep. Most of the recommended procedures are commonsensical. Nevertheless, you should approach the final 24 hours with a conscious sense of strategy, wherein your every move has its reason, as this approach will give you confidence and also ensure that you don't commit any disastrous mental gaffes as a consequence of going about your final preparations less conscientiously.

Among your top priorities on pre-race day, if you have not accomplished it sooner, is to tour the racecourse. The more familiar you can become with a triathlon course before racing on it, the fewer surprises it can throw you. Study the swim course by swimming it, or parts of it, if practical, or from the beach, then slowly drive or ride the bike course, and finally drive, ride, run, or walk the run course (depending on its length). Stop periodically to imagine all that you might be experiencing at this or that particular point in the race, and make strategic notes for your race plan. For example, take note of tough hills and the strength

---

[*] There is no last call in the French Quarter.

and direction of winds, as such factors can and should affect your pacing strategy and possibly even your equipment selection. Later, tour the course again in your imagination at home or wherever you're staying.

If you choose to tour the course without exercising on it, or if you manage to tour it before pre-race day, then one of your top priorities on this day should be an appropriate final workout. Some triathletes prefer not to work out within 24 hours of competing, but many find it to be a good way to stay loose and get rid of some nervous energy that might otherwise keep them awake that night. The workout should be light, though. A 20-minute swim followed by a 20-minute bike ride should do the trick. Otherwise, engage in very little activity on this day, and by all means, stay off your feet and out of the sun, as the former will deaden your legs and the latter will sap your energy. One time I had to work an expo the day before running a marathon. I was on my feet all day—and I was out of the race at mile 18. On the day before my next marathon, my family wanted to visit the zoo. I agreed to join them on one condition: that they literally push me around the zoo in a wheelchair! They did. I had a great race.

The next most important item on your agenda on pre-race day is nutrition. Eat fairly normally, but take in a little more carbohydrate than normal (about 70 percent of your calories) and have your dinner slightly early (6:00 P.M.) if the race start is scheduled for early the next morning. Avoid eating gas-producing foods such as many beans, legumes, and onions. Eating too much fiber before a longer triathlon can also cause mid-race gastrointestinal problems in some triathletes. Ideally, you'll find a traditional pre-race dinner that works well for you and then stay with it, as much for psychological reasons as for physical ones. My personal favorite is fish and rice, or sushi. It burns clean.

Take care of as many logistical and gear-related preparations as possible on this last day, instead of leaving them for race morning. Visit the race expo and pick up your race packet if you do not have it already. Put your bike race number on your bike and/or your bike helmet race number on your helmet and attach your run race number to your race belt. (I like to crumple the number beforehand in order to make it more comfortable and less likely to flap around.) Work out plans for transportation to the race site, seeing your support crew on the course, and so forth. Make sure your transition bag contains everything on your checklist. Shave your legs, if you're into that. Set two alarms. In the evening, after you've taken care of these things, fill the remaining time before you hit the sack with an activity that takes your mind off the race but isn't forced or unduly taxing. Watching a video works for many people. Triathletes frequently make the mistake of turning in too early and then lying awake and staring at the ceiling for a couple hours while they wait for sleep to overtake them. It's better just to accept that you will not get a normal night's sleep on the eve of a race and go to bed only when you're tired. If you've been sleeping well up to this point, getting only five or six hours of shut-eye tonight won't harm you. Mentally rehearse the race a couple more times before you conk out.

The factor that's most likely to determine your wake-up time is the need to eat breakfast early enough so that you don't race on a full stomach. Plan to finish your breakfast no less than two hours, and no more than four hours, before your wave start. Many triathletes find it difficult to eat with a nervous stomach, but even a very light meal is better than none. Eat familiar foods that go down easy. These can include liquids and semisolids, which tend to be favored by triathletes who are prone to a nervous stomach before races. Try to include 200 to 300 grams of carbohydrate and little protein or fat in this meal. I eat the same meal before every race: an energy bar, a banana, a meal replacement shake, and a sports drink. Simply having an automatic breakfast routine that you have confidence in can take you a long way toward overcoming the effect that nerves can have on your stomach. In fact, having a script for every move you make between climbing out of bed and toeing the starting line is a very helpful way to stay calm and focused before a race. Other useful mental techniques include reviewing your goals and race strategy in your mind, engaging in positive self-talk, and listening to music that puts you in the right emotional state for racing.

Upon reaching the race venue, your first order of business (perhaps after getting your body marked) is to set up your transition area. First of all, hop on your bike and make sure everything's working. Set it in the gear in which you'll want to start as you leave the transition area. There's a triathlon held in my area whose course hits you with a brutal climb right out of the transition area. Needless to say, participants who don't pre-set their bikes in their granny gear get off to a horrible start in the second leg of this race. Top off your tires with air and give your bike a final, quick inspection. It's amazing how often even professional triathletes start the bike leg with a leaking tire or loose aerobar. Make sure that your fluid bottles (or alternative hydration system) are filled and in place. Rack your bike so that it's out of the way of your neighbors' bikes (as much as possible) and is easily unracked. Place your helmet upside down on your aerobar or handlebar and place your sunglasses inside it.

Nearly all professional triathletes pre-clip their bike shoes onto the pedals and worry about getting their feet into the shoes once they're on the bike. Once you've mastered it, this is the fastest way to go. The alternative is to place the shoes on a towel in front of your bike (with the straps loosened for easy entry) and clomp your way out of the transition area wearing them (it's illegal to ride your bike in the transition area). Place your running shoes on the towel as well with your number belt, and possibly a running hat or visor, underneath them. Reset your cyclometer, if you have one.

There are three ways you can go with socks. The first option is to wear socks for the bike and run, in which case you'll want to place your socks on top of your cycling shoes if they're not pre-clipped or just on your towel if your shoes are pre-clipped. A second option is to wear socks only for the run, in which case you'll want to place them on top of your running shoes. The third option is to go sockless, as most competitive triathletes choose to do in sprint and middle-distance races. Doing a portion of your training sockless and smearing a thin layer of petroleum jelly on key friction points on the inside of your cycling and running shoes for the race will allow you to do this blister-free. For longer triathlons, socks are recommended. Speaking of friction points, be sure to lubricate any and all areas of your body that may suffer chafing during the race, especially if you're wearing a wetsuit. And don't forget to apply sunscreen as well.

If you'll be using gels or energy bars during the race, you can either swim with them in the rear pocket of your triathlon suit, if you're wearing a wetsuit over it, or place them in your helmet and then stuff them in your rear pocket during your first transition. You can also mold unwrapped energy bars to the top tube of your bike. Lastly, learn a lesson from poor Jim and trace the route you will take when entering the transition area and finding your transition spot from the swim and bike legs so that you can do the same without any wasted time in the race itself. Take note of landmarks and even count bike racks if that will help.

The next order of business is your pre-race warm-up. Like breakfast, the pre-race warm-up is an important activity that many triathletes give short shrift due to nervousness. This is not only unfortunate but also ironic, because warming up is a great way to channel nervous energy and restore some degree of calm. It also prepares your body for the coming race effort and thereby helps you perform better than you could do without a warm-up. Ideally, your warm-up should include a little cycling, a little running, a little stretching, and a little swimming, in this order. The length of your warm-up should vary inversely in proportion to the length of the race. Before a sprint triathlon, try to spend a good 40 minutes warming up. Before an Iron-distance event, 15 minutes of swimming and

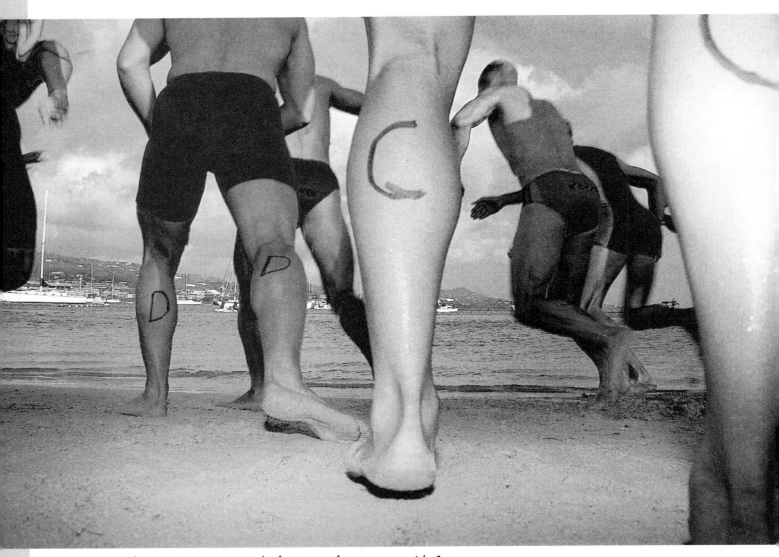

Try to complete your pre-race warm-up within five minutes of your wave start. *John Segesta*

stretching will do. Keep the intensity very low, except for three or four swim sprints lasting perhaps 20 seconds each that you perform at the very end of the warm-up. If possible, time your warm-up to end within five minutes of your wave start.

Another major agenda item on race morning is using the bathroom, early and often. Simply put, you will want to use the bathroom as frequently as possible, and give yourself every possible opportunity to use the bathroom, between the time you wake up and the time you start. You don't want the dead weight and you don't want to be troubled by bathroom urges during a race.* To some degree, you just have to hope your body will be ready to void first thing race morning. With time, your body should come to know when it is about to race and will become very accommodating with respect to your need for empty bowels and bladder at such times. (Veteran triathletes bring a whole new meaning to the term "potty training.") You'll also want to develop a knack for avoiding the interminable waits that can develop for the portable toilets at the race site. Tactics I've used with success include visiting the woods (for number one only), having my support crew hold a place in line for me, and finding an out-of-the-way toilet along my warm-up route. Besides practice, two measures that can help you achieve your "ideal race weight" on race morning are taking a dose of caffeine (a diuretic) and terminating all fluid intake between 30 minutes and 5 minutes before your wave start.

As for last-minute fueling, try to take in 16 to 24 ounces of water and sports drink in the two hours preceding your half-hour fluid intake cut-off and a few more ounces of sports drink about 5 minutes before your wave start. You may also wish to consume an energy gel at this time.

The Race Itself

The swim start is one of the most critical moments in any triathlon for triathletes of every level. It is the most chaotic and uncontrollable portion of the race, and also the most uncharacteristic in terms of the nature of triathlon itself. Anaerobic and often rather violent, it's more like a football play than an endurance race. Your primary objectives in the swim start are to get through the surf (if there is any) efficiently, to pick the best line toward the first buoy, and to avoid bumping into other triathletes. If you're competitive, try to start toward the front and get out

---

*The exceptions are long-distance triathlons, wherein it is normal to stop (or not stop!) and urinate one or more times "on the clock."

fast. By practicing sprints in training, you can cultivate the ability to recover from this hard, initial effort after easing back into your race pace some 100 or 200 yards into the race. If you're a slow swimmer, start at the back or toward either side and begin slowly to avoid crowding and jostling, which might put you in a panic. When picking your line, try to account for the direction of the current.

If possible, draft behind other swimmers throughout the swim portion of the triathlon. While drafting on the bike is illegal for most competitors in most races, drafting in the swim is not only legal but just plain smart, as it reduces the energy expenditure required to maintain a given pace. The ideal candidate for drafting is a swimmer who's swimming just slightly faster than your own pace. Don't make it your first priority to find such a swimmer, because it requires a degree of coincidence, but don't pass up opportunities that present themselves, either. If another swimmer should happen to pass you gradually at any point during the swim, slip behind him or her and follow along at a distance of a foot or two. Don't allow yourself to get dragged along by a much stronger swimmer or get bogged down by one who's flagging. Swim your own race at your own pace, utilizing the presence of others only when, and as long as, it works to your benefit.

Pacing is one of the most important aspects of race execution in all three legs of a triathlon. Good pacing is all about expending energy as evenly as possible throughout a race and at a rate that allows you to finish just before reaching a level of carbohydrate depletion that brings with it a substantial drop in performance. Racing at a perfectly consistent pace throughout any leg of a triathlon is not possible. Variations in the course and environment (hills, turns, winds, currents), changes in how you feel, and mental factors all cause pace and energy output to vary. Nevertheless, a more or less even expenditure of energy is the ideal. Pacing is an art that one can never perfect, but can always improve upon. The greatest improvements in one's instinct for pacing—and it is a cultivated instinct—come through race experience. Have you ever watched youngsters do their first one-mile fun run? Ninety percent of them take off sprinting, and find themselves reduced to a death march 100 yards later. In their next fun run, most of these kids (not all of them!) will know better, and will accordingly hold back in a conscious effort to run the entire distance at an even pace. Triathletes usually go through a less extreme, and sometimes inverted, version of the same process. Some new triathletes bonk before reaching the finish line, while others finish knowing they could have gone a little faster, or perhaps a lot faster. In either case, they can take this information, along with knowledge of what this effort felt like and the actual numerical pace they maintained in each segment of the race, and apply it in the next race with a view toward optimizing their energy expenditure. What complicates this process a bit is the fact that race pace is different for different race distances, and to a lesser extent for different courses of the same distance.

You can rely on objective gauges (cyclometer, sports watch) to some degree to control your pace in the bike and run portions of a race, but the main gauge must be signals from your own body. By performing a certain amount of your training in all three disciplines at your anticipated race pace (for one or more race distances), you can teach your body what it feels like and you will then be more likely to set off at this pace in each leg of the races themselves. At the same time, you can also use training times and splits and perceived exertion in workouts of various intensities to determine appropriate race pace—and for that matter, to set goals—for upcoming races.

Fast transitions are another important component of good race execution. The swim-bike transition (T1) is generally the more critical one. Always continue swimming until your hands touch sandy bottom. Standing any earlier will result in an agonizingly slow wade to shore. While running from the beach to transition, remove your goggles and swim cap and remove the upper half of your body from your wetsuit, if you're wearing one. There's no single right way to perform your transition, but no matter how you do it, move deliberately and efficiently, rather than hastily. It's the hasty that end up sitting on the pavement trying desperately to yank their feet out of the inside-out ankle cuffs of their wetsuit. The order of your movements should be rote, as you will be semidelirious at this point in the race. When approaching the transition area on your bike (T2), it's a good idea to stand out of the saddle and stretch your legs a bit in anticipation of the run. You may lose a few seconds in doing this but these seconds will be more than made up for in the first mile of the run, as your pre-loosened hamstrings will have a lesser adjustment to make.

Two further important facets of race execution that I'll discuss in greater detail in later chapters are the mental and nutritional facets. Speaking generally, I'll say here that the cliché holds: Racing is at least 50 percent mental. A triathlete thinks all the way through a triathlon. Maintaining control over the unbroken internal monologue that takes place during the race experience is critical to successful racing. Intelligent fueling and hydration, meanwhile, are equally critical with respect to the physical 50 percent of racing. Getting through a triathlon without taking in the right nutrients in the right proportions is like trying to complete the Indy 500 without pit stops.

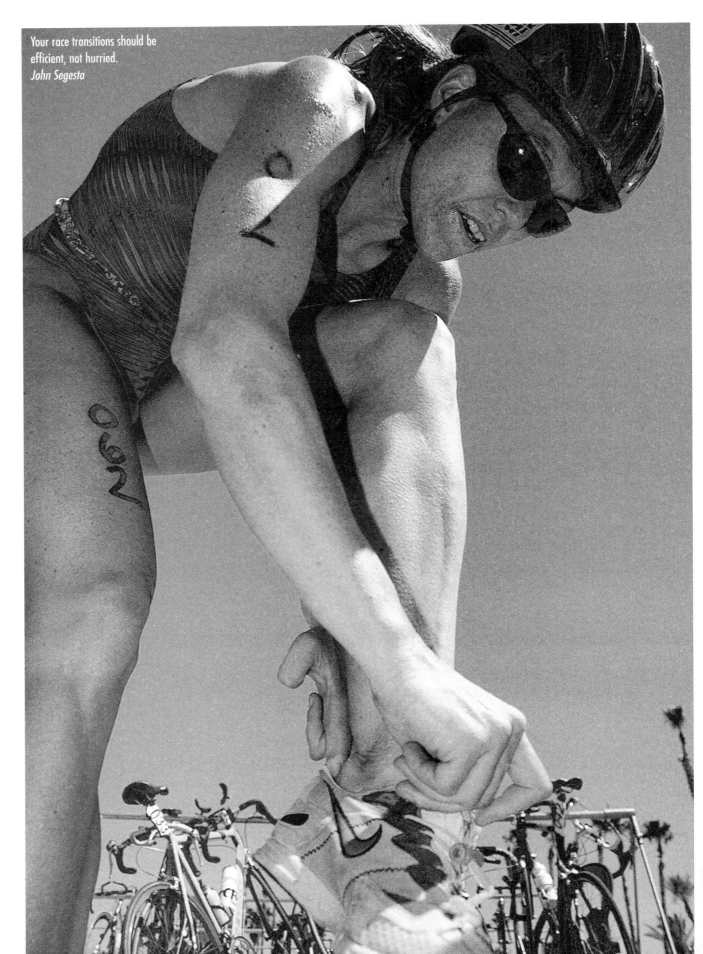

Your race transitions should be
efficient, not hurried.
John Segesta

One Final Point

I began this chapter with a story that demonstrated how a person should not race a triathlon—in a word, without forethought. I'd like to conclude this chapter with another story, which demonstrates the right way to race.

Many years ago, at a sprint triathlon held in Santa Barbara, legendary age-grouper Pete Kain arrived at T2 holding second place overall, only to discover that his racing flats were missing. Failing to discover them in the immediate vicinity of his transition spot and feeling the pressure of time, Kain made a decision. He decided to run barefoot. After all, the run course was only four miles long. So, he set off barefoot, which was fine at first, because the run began on grass. But then he hit pavement, and within a minute of this Kain found himself in greater pain than he could ignore. At this point he was approaching an adolescent race volunteer directing race traffic at an intersection. "What size shoe do you wear?" Kain called out to the boy. "Nine and a half," he replied, taken aback. "Close enough," said Kain, who wore an eleven and a half. After extracting a promise of their return, the volunteer gave Kain his shoes, into which the desperate triathlete hastily crammed his feet, and he resumed running. Despite the delay, Kain was not passed by a single competitor.

The lesson? No matter how much you plan and prepare for a triathlon, at least one unexpected event will happen within it, guaranteed. And when the unexpected does happen, you just have to keep your hand away from the panic button and roll with it. You can't control everything that happens in a race, but you can control your reactions. Some amount of improvisation will be required of you in every triathlon you ever do. The more calmly and creatively you're able to address unexpected happenings, and the less you let them bother you, the more successful you will be.

Triathlon Vacations

One of the things I miss most about working as a staff editor with *Triathlete* is the travel. An important part of the job of a *Triathlete* editor is to travel around the world and watch very healthy people exercise on and around lovely beaches under blue skies. I myself visited New Orleans, Hawaii, Saint Maarten, Brazil, and Argentina, to name just a few locations, for the purpose of watching men and women practice my favorite sport, and on a few occasions I was actually able to participate in the very races I was present to cover.

I came away from this experience feeling pretty well convinced that there are few better excuses and focal points for a vacation than participation in a triathlon. First-rate triathlons are held in dozens of the world's most worthy places to visit, from Switzerland to the Southeast Asian island of Laguna Phuket. When you visit such places to compete in a triathlon, you have the opportunity to be more than just a typical tourist there, but instead to participate in creating one of the area's big events. Also, rather than experiencing a tourist's isolation, you arrive into a community of like-minded people with whom making friends—sometimes lifelong friends—is relatively easy. And last but not least, you don't come home from such vacations in worse shape than you left in, as one does from most vacations!

There are a few different ways you can proceed in terms of choosing a triathlon around which to plan a vacation. The first option is to choose a place you'd like to visit and then look into whether any good triathlons are held there. A second option is to peruse the race calendar at the back of each issue of *Triathlete* and see what catches your eye. A third option is to solicit recommendations from fellow triathletes. Indeed, whichever option you begin with, it's always best if you can talk to at least one person who's done the race you're interested in doing, first of all for an evaluation, and later, once you've made a decision, for useful information about how to plan for it. If you don't personally know anyone who's done the race you'd like to do, you can find such people on the Internet through newsgroups like rec.sport.triathlon.

It's a good idea not to travel far for a triathlon you know little about. Established and well-known events typically have the highest levels of participant satisfaction. On the other hand, some smaller and more out-of-the-way events are quite wonderful and their organizers often bend over backward to please foreign travelers. In many cases you can communicate directly with the directors of such races, and there's no better way to get a sense of whether the triathlon is worth committing to.

Another important consideration is this: Do you show up early and do your touring before the race or stay over and tour afterward? Here's my advice: If you'd like to tour a fairly broad area and not just the immediate vicinity of the race city, do your touring afterward, as it will be difficult in such a case to perform workouts and take care of race preparations. If you don't plan to stray far, arriving early is preferable, as it allows you to get comfortable in your surroundings, prepare without haste, and participate fully in the whole scene that precedes the race itself. An exception is the case where you're interested in really partying, which is best done after you've gotten your triathlon out of the way.

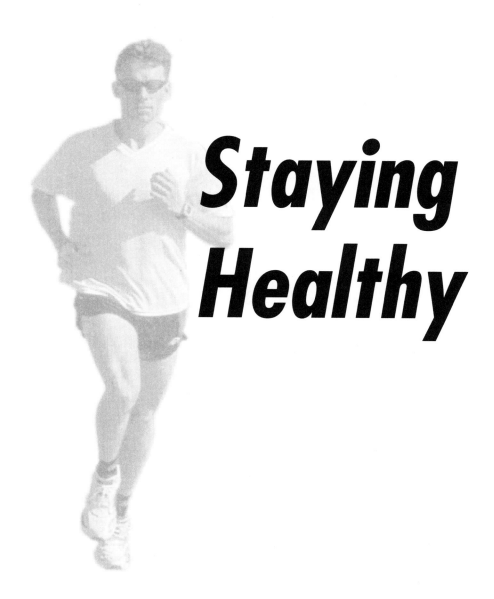

CHAPTER 8

Staying Healthy

The triathlete's lifestyle is not without its risks. For example, there is a vanishingly small but nevertheless real chance that, during the swim portion of a triathlon, you could be knocked silly by a surfacing military submarine. However, this chapter is not about handling such bizarre twists of fate as these. Rather, it deals with the most common unintended side effects of triathlon training: orthopedic injury, viral infections, and general fatigue.

It's weird. Frequent, hard exercise makes one both more *and* less prone to illness and injury. On the one hand, it generally strengthens the musculoskeletal and immune systems, but on the other hand it can also be directly or indirectly responsible for individual instances of sickness, joint malfunction, and tissue breakdown. And while triathlon training should increase your overall vitality, doing too much training in combination with everything else you do on a daily basis can leave you run-down. The goal of this chapter is to give you the knowledge you'll need to minimize the likelihood of your experiencing these problems and to recover from them quickly when they cannot be prevented. Let's begin with injury prevention.

Preventing Injuries

We humans are not celebrated for our foresight. Generally, we'd rather *react* than *act*. In this regard, triathletes are no different than others. This is why few triathletes practice proper injury prevention techniques, and why overuse injuries are so common among triathletes. I'm a case in point. I developed all eight of the overuse injuries I will discuss later in this chapter, plus a few extras, before I finally woke up and began to consistently practice the following methods of injury prevention. I strongly recommend that you begin to practice any of these methods you're not practicing already, *today,* so that you may spare yourself from experiencing any of the eight common overuse injuries (and various less common ones) you have not experienced already.

Rest

Workouts cause dehydration, carbohydrate fuel depletion, metabolic waste buildup, muscle tissue trauma, muscle protein breakdown, and other effects from which the body must recover before the next workout occurs. Rest is the primary condition of this reversal. Insufficient rest can lead to poor workouts, stagnating fitness, injury, illness, and chronic fatigue.

On the other hand, getting too much rest is also undesirable. If you don't train hard and consistently, you'll probably remain healthy, but you won't get very fit. So the goal is to get just enough rest. But this objective tends to carry with it a greater risk of resting too little than too much—after all, how else can you determine the limit of how much training you can handle except by crossing it?

For this reason, and because the consequences of slightly undertraining are not as detrimental as those of slightly overtraining, I encourage you to err on the side of getting a little more rest than you may need, at least until you've become adept at interpreting your body's needs and can truly ride the limit. By planning your training sensibly, according to the guidelines I've shared in preceding chapters, you can get sufficient rest without sacrificing fitness. And if ever you do encounter a period in your training when you feel persistently flat, caution becomes the better half of valor. Retreat is prudent. Skip or shorten a workout, or even treat yourself to an unscheduled recovery week. Doing so just might save you from having to rest much more in the near future.

Massage

You can't beat a sports massage for injury prevention that you can *feel*. While not as pleasurable as your typical spa massage, a good sports massage certainly has its moments, and it will leave you feeling like new afterward. For this reason, nearly every elite endurance athlete now swears by this recovery technique, and a growing number of age-groupers are following their example.

Sports massage enhances recovery and helps prevent injuries in several ways. The most important effect of massage with respect to recovery is that it substantially increases blood circulation to the muscles and keeps it elevated for as long as an hour afterward. This extra blood flow flushes metabolic wastes from the muscles, hurries in nutrients that repair muscle damage, and controls inflammation and the pain associated with it.

Massage also alleviates muscular trigger points (areas of sensitivity), mobilizes adhesions, and breaks up scar tissue in the muscles, restoring normal function. And some believe it even enhances the electrical flow of signals between the brain and muscle nerves, which improves the functioning of motor units.

Yet another use for massage is identifying incipient injuries before they become painful during exercise, as well as muscle imbalances that could lead to injury and are probably compromising your technique and efficiency. For this you'll need a massage therapist with an interest in endurance sports and a lot of experience in working with endurance athletes. Solicit your therapist's assessment of the condition of your important muscles and tendons and ask him or her to point out left side–right side asymmetries.

The bad news about sports massage is that you can expect to pay $40 to $80 for a one-hour massage from a skilled professional. If money's no object and you're serious about performance, schedule one session per week, at least during the build and peak phases of your training cycles. Otherwise, you can compromise by getting half-body sessions or spacing them out more (say, once a month). There are also various self-massage techniques that you can and should practice, which you can learn from a number of available books and videos on the subject. If used properly, devices like the foam rollers used by physical therapists can yield some of the same benefits as sports massage, such as releasing trigger points.

Stretching

Triathletes do not need to be more flexible than the average person. In fact, highly flexible triathletes are likely to be less efficient, especially when running, than triathletes who have only a normal range of motion at the major joints. If you can raise your arm straight over your head, you're flexible enough to be a world-class swimmer. If you can raise your knee to the height of your navel when standing, you are flexible enough to win the Tour de France or to break the marathon world record.

Does this mean a triathlete should never engage in flexibility exercises? It does not. To the contrary, all triathletes should regularly stretch certain muscles, because the repetitive contractions that the hardest-working muscles (called *prime movers)* undergo in training tend to reduce the elasticity of these muscles (i.e., tighten them), leaving them susceptible to tearing. Muscles that play a secondary role in the same movement patterns, called *synergists,* also have a tendency to tighten up, as do certain *postural muscles* that hold a contracted position throughout the performance of a given activity. But the tightening of prime movers, synergists, and postural muscles does not happen in isolation. Whenever a major working muscle becomes tightened through repetition, one or more muscles on the opposite side of the same joint (called *antagonists*), whose main job is to stabilize the joint, tend to become weakened and overstretched, as can other stabilizer muscles near the moving joint. The resulting muscle imbalance can cause instability in the affected joint and eventually dysfunction. It can also cause changes in technique that can in turn lead to dysfunction in other parts of the body.

For example, consider the repetitive arm motions involved in freestyle swimming. Here, big, powerful muscles of the chest and back serve as the prime movers while a group of smaller back muscles known collectively as scapular stabilizers, and a group of internal shoulder muscles called the rotator cuff, bear the primary responsibility for stabilizing the shoulder. But because the job of moving the arm is so much more demanding than that of stabilizing the shoulder, the prime mover muscles become strong and begin to help with stabilization, leaving the stabilizers with even less to do. But a prime mover cannot ever do the job of stabilization as well as an adequately conditioned group of stabilizers. So, the more the swimmer swims, and the lazier the scapular stabilizers get, the less stable the shoulder gets. This can and often does result in tissue damage and dysfunction deep inside the shoulder joint.

Stretching the prime movers is half of what is needed to prevent or undo such problems. The other half, which I'll discuss in the next section, is strengthening the antagonists and other stabilizers.[*] Strengthening the prime movers and synergists through a wider range of motion than they normally go through in swimming, cycling, and running is also helpful.

---

[*] I wish to clarify that no muscle is always a prime mover, antagonist, synergist, or stabilizer. In fact, in cyclical movements such as those performed in swimming, cycling, and running, most of the involved muscles serve different functions in different phases. For example, the hamstrings function as antagonists during the thigh-lift portion of the running stride, but they act as prime movers during the toe-off portion. But each muscle has a primary role in a given type of activity (the hamstrings are primarily a prime mover in running), and that's what I'm focusing on in this discussion.

Muscles that tend to become too tight in triathletes are those of the calf, the hamstrings, the hip flexors, the internal shoulder rotators, the neck extensors, and the chest muscles. All act as prime movers and synergists in the triathlon disciplines except the neck muscles, which become tight from maintaining a contracted posture during swimming and cycling. Two major tendons, the iliotibial band and the Achilles tendon, also tend to become tight. You should stretch all of these muscles and tendons daily. The best time to stretch is anytime. Some people like to stretch early in the morning, others before bed. You make the call. As long as you do a proper warm-up, it is not necessary to stretch before a workout unless you have a problem muscle that requires it. Immediately after a workout is an ideal time to stretch, because you've just done what stretching is meant, in a sense, to undo. Following is a set of stretching exercises designed to lengthen muscles that tend to become tight through triathlon training.

NECK STRETCH

Put your hands behind your head and splay your elbows wide, prisoner-style. Tip your head forward and apply a little downward pressure with your hands. Hold the stretch for 10 or 12 seconds and relax. Turn your head slightly to the left and stretch again. Now stretch the other side. Repeat all three stretches once or twice.

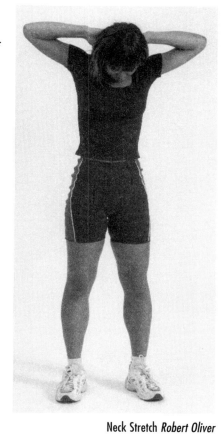

Neck Stretch *Robert Oliver*

CHEST AND SHOULDER STRETCH

Stand comfortably and place your hands about three feet apart along a length of resistance band or some other kind of elastic strap or cable. Use an overhand grip. Inhale and lift both arms directly over your head. Exhale and carry the strap behind your back in a smooth arc, without bending your elbows, and stopping when the strap is at roughly the height of your diaphragm. Reach as far behind you as possible. You should feel a nice stretch in your shoulders and chest. Inhale and lift your arms back over your head. Exhale and return to the start position. Do this three times more.

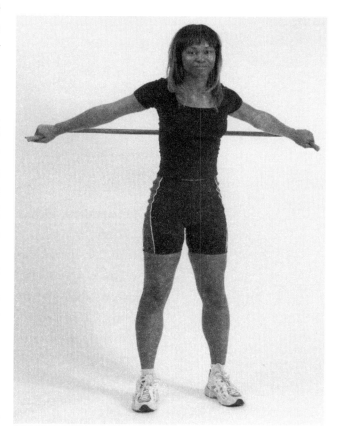

Chest and Shoulder Stretch *Robert Oliver*

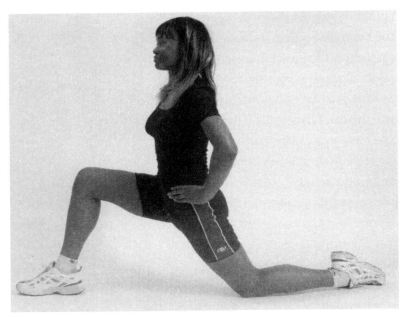

Lunge Stretch *Robert Oliver*

LUNGE STRETCH

Kneel on your right knee and place your left foot on the floor well in front of your body. Draw your navel toward your spine and roll your pelvis backward. Now put your weight forward into the lunge until you feel a good stretch in your right hip flexors (located where your thigh joins your pelvis). You can enhance the stretch by raising your right arm over your head and bending to the left. Hold the stretch for 20 seconds and then repeat on the left side.

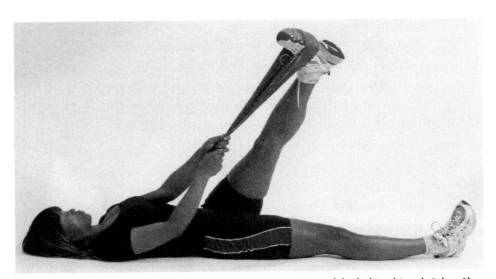

Hamstring, Hip, and Iliotibial Band Stretch *Robert Oliver*

HAMSTRING, HIP, AND ILIOTIBIAL BAND STRETCH

Lie on your back and loop a strap around the arch of your right foot. Hold the strap in your left hand and extend your right arm away from your torso along the floor. Straighten your leg as much as possible and flex your ankle (i.e., bring your toes toward you). Grasp the strap at the highest point possible without allowing your left shoulder blade to lose contact with the floor. Exhale and swing your right leg straight across your body, bringing your heel as close to the floor as you can without twisting any other part of your body. (You may find that you can't go very far!) Inhale and return to the top. Do this three times more and then switch legs.

TWO-WAY CALF STRETCH

Stand with a thick book or other solid object wedged under the ball of your right foot so that this foot is angled upward 30 to 60 degrees (enough that you can feel a stretch). Hold this stretch for 20 seconds. This will stretch the gastrocnemius, which is the larger, more visible muscle in your calf. Now bend your knee slightly and feel the stretch migrate downward into your soleus muscle. Hold this stretch for 20 seconds. Now stretch the right side.

ACHILLES TENDON STRETCH

Stand in a split stance, one foot a step ahead of the other, with both feet flat on the ground and both knees slightly bent. Now bend your back leg a little more and concentrate on trying to sink your butt straight down toward the heel of that foot. Keep your torso upright. You should begin to feel a stretch in your Achilles tendon. You may have to fiddle with your position before you find it. When you do, hold it for 10 or 12 seconds, relax, and then stretch it a couple more times.

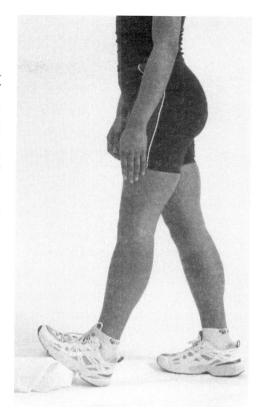

Calf Stretch, step one (gastrocnemius) *Robert Oliver*

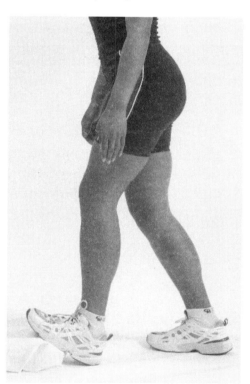

Calf Stretch, step two (soleus) *Robert Oliver*

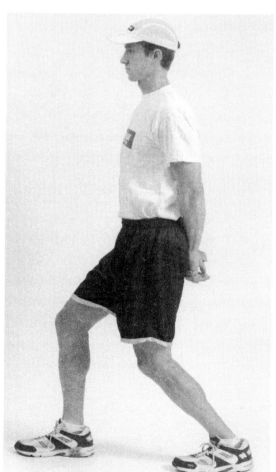

Achilles Tendon Stretch *Robert Oliver*

185

Strength Training

Muscle weakness is a factor in a majority of overuse injuries. I mentioned the relationship between weak scapular stabilizers and rotator cuff muscles and swimmer's shoulder already. Running and cycling injuries often have a similar etiology. In running, for example, the calf muscles are prime movers while their antagonists on the medial and frontal sides of the shin act as stabilizers. However, heavy repetition leads to overdevelopment of the calf muscles relative to their antagonists and leaves the latter unable to properly stabilize the ankle. This instability, in turn, can allow the foot to overpronate, and overpronation frequently results in the overuse injuries known as runner's knee, Achilles tendinitis, and plantar fasciitis.

In cycling, the muscles of the lower back bear the main burden of supporting a sharply bent trunk. The lower abdominals are supposed to help, but these muscles tend to be weak and lazy in denizens of our sitting-centered society, so they really don't help. The ultimate consequence is overstretching and tearing of muscles in the lower back, accompanied by debilitating pain.

The primary purpose of strength training for triathletes is to correct the muscle imbalances that swimming, cycling, and running, not to mention sitting, tend to foster. The muscles that are typically underdeveloped in triathletes are the medial and frontal shin muscles, the hip abductors, the gluteal muscles, the abdominals, the scapular stabilizers, and the rotator cuff muscles, all of which every triathlete should proactively strengthen with resistance exercise. However, these are not the only muscles that triathletes should strengthen, and here's why. There is a secondary purpose of strength training for triathletes, unrelated to injury prevention, which is to increase one's ability to generate power in the swimming, cycling, and running movement patterns.

Whereas being unusually flexible is no advantage for triathletes, being strong (in particular movement patterns) is another story. Given two cyclists with matching VO_2 maximums and matching levels of energy economy, the faster of the two will be the cyclist with stronger leg (and gluteal) muscles. It simply takes more strength to pedal faster. And the same rule applies in swimming and running. Also, in swimming and running especially, but in cycling as well, forces used in forward propulsion are transferred between the upper body and legs through the trunk, and so there is an advantage in developing a reserve of strength in this area, too.

The strength training method that is most familiar to us is the bodybuilding method. But as a triathlete, you should not strength train like a bodybuilder. Bodybuilders train muscles. They perform exercises that isolate and concentrate force upon individual muscles as much as possible. The result is big muscles that look powerful but are virtually incapable of cooperating with other muscles to perform athletic movements. Triathletes must train movements, not individual muscles. A majority of the exercises you perform should simulate and intensify some action that your body performs in swimming, cycling, or running, because your goal is to make your stabilizers better able to stabilize *during swimming, cycling, and running,* and to make your prime movers and synergists better able to generate force *during swimming, cycling, and running.* In other words, these exercises must be *functional.*

A classic bodybuilding exercise like the Barbell Bench Press, with its full trunk stabilization, muscular isolation, and symmetrical limb movements, simulates nothing you'll ever do in the water, on the bike, or in running shoes. Functional strength training is all about training your body to perform sport-specific movements with correct form and greater force. Like swimming, cycling, and running themselves, your key strength-training exercises should involve balance and trunk (or core) stabilization, independent limb movements, and cooperation among several muscles that are centrally involved in the swimming and pedaling strokes and the running stride. Here is a full-body functional strength workout for triathletes:

Strength Workout for Triathletes

This workout is designed to correct the muscular imbalances that are common in triathletes and to improve power in swimming, cycling, and running. It is meant to be performed year-round, but includes just six exercises and requires minimal time. During the off-season, pre-base period, and perhaps also the first half of the base phase of training, do the workout two to three times a week and perform two to three sets of each exercise in a circuit. During the remainder of the training cycle, do the workout twice a week and perform one to three sets of each exercise in a circuit.

The workout requires a stability ball and a set of resistance bands. Stability balls cost $30 to $50 and they come in various sizes, so make sure you get the right size for your height. Your fitness equipment retailer can help you. Resistance bands are basically a length of surgical tubing with handles on either end. They come in various degrees of thickness and/or tension for various degrees of resistance. I recommend getting two bands for the sake of versatility. Tell your fitness equipment

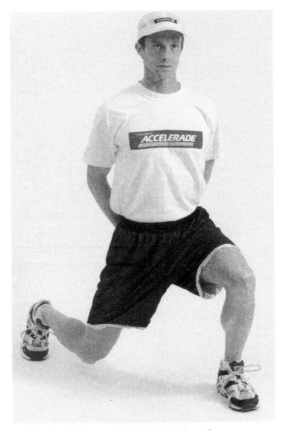

Multidirectional Lunge and Heel Raise *Robert Oliver*

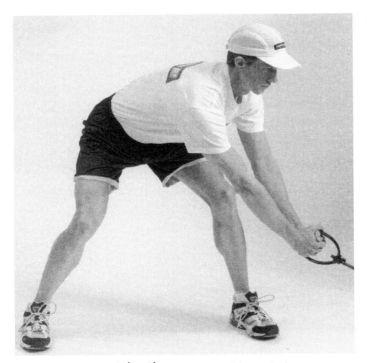

Two Arm Twist, step one *Robert Oliver*

retailer how you plan to use your bands and, frankly, about how strong you are, and he or she should be able to match you up with the right ones. This will set you back no more than $20 to $40. When choosing resistance bands, be sure to get ones that have a door attachment. Alternatively, you can use a cable pulley station at a gym.

MULTIDIRECTIONAL LUNGE AND HEEL RAISE

Benefits: This exercise strengthens virtually all of the muscles below the waist, corrects muscular imbalances in the hips and thighs, and improves cycling and running power.

Procedure: Stand comfortably with your right hand holding your left wrist behind your back. Take a moderately large step forward with your left foot and dip downward until the knee of the rear leg almost touches the floor. Keep your torso upright. Press back upright and step backward to the start position. Next lunge 45 degrees to the left of forward with the same foot and return again to the start position. Lunge three more times: straight to the left, 45 degrees to the rear, and finally straight back, returning to the start position after each lunge. Now repeat the same pattern of five lunges with the right leg. Finally, return to the start position and perform 15 to 20 heel raises, lifting your heels as far above the floor as possible, pausing briefly, and lowering your heels again slowly.

To make this exercise more challenging, you can perform it holding dumbbells at your sides or a weighted barbell on your upper back.

TWO ARM TWIST

Benefits: This exercise strengthens the chest, rotator cuff, scapular stabilizers, obliques, and hip abductors, corrects muscular imbalances in the shoulder girdle, trunk, and pelvis, and enhances core stability.

Procedure: Attach a resistance band to a door at ankle height. Stand in a wide stance with your left side facing the door and most of your weight on the inside foot. Bend forward slightly at the waist and begin by holding the handle in both hands just outside your left shin. Using both arms, pull the cable upward and across your body, beginning outside your left ankle and finishing above your right shoulder, and rotating your trunk as you go. Return smoothly to the start position. Do 12 to 15 repetitions and then switch sides.

HIP LIFT AND HAMSTRING CURL

Benefits: This exercise strengthens the abdominals, glutes, and hamstrings, corrects muscular imbalances in the trunk and pelvis, and improves power in cycling, running, and the swim kick.

Procedure: Lie face up on the floor and rest your heels on a stability ball, with your legs straight. Rest your arms at your sides, palms down. Lift your hips up toward the ceiling by contracting your abdominals and butt. When your body forms a straight line from neck to heels, bend your knees and pull the ball toward your butt. Extend your legs again and then lower your butt back to the floor. Do 10 to 20 repetitions.

To make this exercise more challenging (a lot more challenging!), rest just one heel on the ball and elevate the other heel a few inches above it. Perform the complete exercise with just one leg and then do it again with the other.

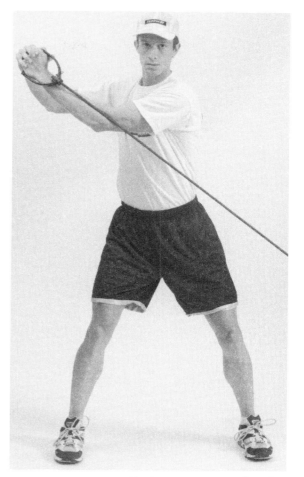

Two Arm Twist, step two *Robert Oliver*

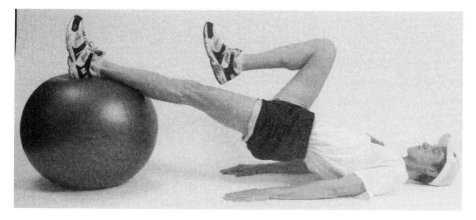

Hip Lift and Hamstring Curl
Robert Oliver

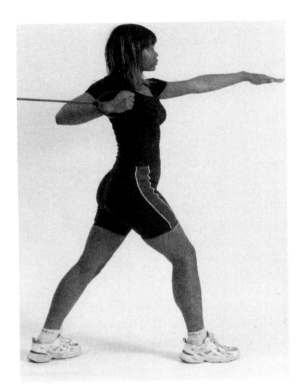

Single Arm Push, step one *Robert Oliver*

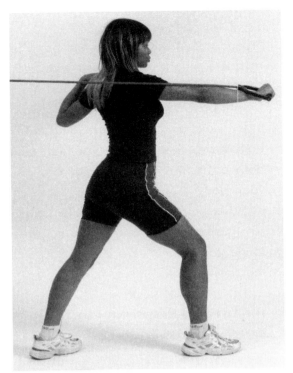

Single Arm Push, step two *Robert Oliver*

SINGLE ARM PUSH

Benefits: This exercise strengthens the chest, anterior deltoids, and obliques, and improves swimming arm cycle power and core stability.

Procedure: Attach a resistance band to a door slightly above shoulder height. Stand in a split stance, facing away from the resistance, with most of your weight on your rear foot. Hold the cable handle against your chest in your right hand and reach forward with your left arm. Throw a smooth, controlled jab. Initiate the movement from the hips, then twist the trunk and finally move the arms. As you push with one arm, retract the other. Repeat for 30 seconds and then switch arms.

SINGLE ARM PULL

Benefits: This exercise strengthens the scapular stabilizers and obliques, corrects muscular imbalances in the shoulder girdle, improves power in the arm cycle in swimming and the arm swing in running, and enhances core stability.

Procedure: Attach a resistance band to a door slightly above shoulder height. Stand in a split stance, facing toward the resistance, with most of your weight on your forward foot. Hold the cable handle in either hand at full forward reach. Pull the handle toward your armpit. Initiate the movement from the hips, then twist the trunk and finally move the arms. As you retract the pulling arm, reach forward with the other. Repeat for 30 seconds and then switch arms.

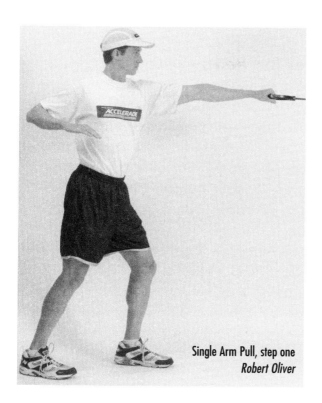

Single Arm Pull, step one
Robert Oliver

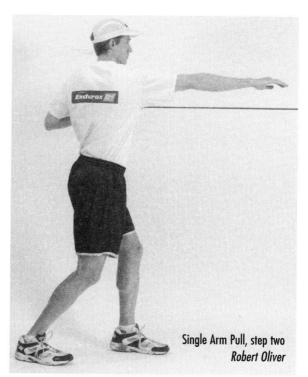

Single Arm Pull, step two
Robert Oliver

FORWARD ROLL

Benefits: This exercise strengthens the rotator cuff, scapular stabilizers, and abdominals, and corrects imbalances in the shoulder girdle and trunk.

Procedure: Kneel on the floor facing the ball, lean forward slightly, and place your forearms on top of the ball with your fingers interlaced. Pull your belly button toward your spine. Slowly roll the ball forward by extending your forearms out in front of you and allowing your body to tilt toward the floor. Concentrate on maintaining perfect alignment of your spine. Stop just before you're forced to arch your back. Hold this position for three seconds and then return to the start position, exhaling as you do so. Do up to 12 repetitions.

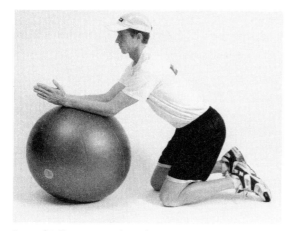

Forward Roll, step one *Robert Oliver*

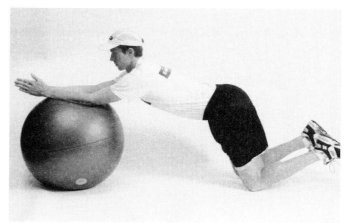

Forward Roll, step two *Robert Oliver*

Corrective Exercises for the Lower Leg

If you could choose only one muscle area to strengthen, it should be your calf muscles' antagonists on the medial and anterior sides of the shin. Doing so will stabilize your ankles and reduce strain on your calf muscles during running, and can help to correct overpronation, thus preventing running injuries associated with ankle instability and over-pronation. It will also increase your running efficiency by lessening ground contact time and increasing the amount of force that returns to your foot from the ground.

Some of the following exercises strengthen muscles in the foot as well as muscles in the shin. The foot muscles actually do quite a bit of work during the contact phase of the running stride. When these muscles are strong, they get your foot back off the ground more quickly and are able to push off more powerfully. They're worth paying attention to.

TOE DIP

Stand on a block or sturdy box with your heels supported and your forefeet hanging over the edge. Hold on to a wall for support. Lower your toes toward the floor as far as comfortably possible and then lift them again. Repeat for 30 seconds.

PILLOW BALANCING

Place a pillow on the floor and balance on it with one shoeless foot for 30 seconds, and then balance on the other foot, and repeat. At first it will be difficult to last 30 seconds, but you'll quickly improve. Keep it challenging by using a bigger or softer pillow, by stacking pillows, and/or by balancing longer.

TOWEL SCRUNCH

Sit in a chair with your feet flat on the floor and a towel laid out just in front of your toes. Use the toes of both feet to pull (or scrunch) the towel underneath your feet bit by bit. Pull once with the left foot, then once with the right, and continue. This is much easier on a wood or tile floor than on a carpeted one.

PICKING UP MARBLES

Sit in a chair and use the toes of both feet to repeatedly pick up marbles from the floor and drop them down again. Do this for a few minutes.

TRACING THE ALPHABET

While sitting in a chair, lift your left foot a few inches above the floor and trace each letter of the alphabet in the air, as though your big toe were a piece of chalk. After you trace Z, switch to the right foot.

Dealing with Injuries

When you begin to experience recurring pain in any part of your body during or following workouts, follow this five-step protocol for dealing with overuse injuries of all types.

1. Modify Your Training

The majority of overuse injuries that befall triathletes are painful and debilitating only in the mode in which they were caused (usually running), which makes working around them and maintaining fitness in spite of them fairly easy. For example, plantar fasciitis, which is associated with running, will not hinder swimming or cycling in the least. So, unless the injury you've developed is of a sort that clearly calls for complete rest, try to modify your training to work around whatever problem you're having, either by reducing training volume in the affected discipline or ceasing to train in the affected discipline and taking up the slack in the others.

In some cases, you can work around an injury even within the affected discipline. For example, when suffering from shin splints or plantar fasciitis, you might be able to run on grass, sand, or a treadmill, although not on pavement.

2. Reduce Inflammation

Tissue inflammation accompanies all overuse injuries. In fact, the pain you feel when an overuse condition develops is generally caused less by the injury itself than by the tissue inflammation that develops in the area of the injury as the body tries to heal itself. While treating the symptoms of pain and inflammation alone solves nothing, it is a very helpful measure to take in conjunction with measures aimed at dealing with the underlying problem.

The key is to act aggressively. Ice the affected area not once or twice a day, but three or four times, at least. Massage it regularly with a heat-inducing cream such as Tiger Balm. Take the maximum recommended daily dosage of aspirin or ibuprofen, or better yet, get your hands on a prescription anti-inflammatory. And if the injury exists in an area that you can compress with a compression bandage, try this as well. Some triathletes have good luck with acupuncture, too, although Western medical practitioners don't know why.

3. Diagnose the Problem

In most cases, you can diagnose your overuse injury on your own, because the vast majority of injuries triathletes experience represent one of just eight easily distinguished types: swimmer's shoulder, lower back pain, runner's knee, hamstring strain, iliotibial band syndrome, shin splints, Achilles tendinitis, and plantar fasciitis (all of which are described in the next section). While the specific diagnosis has little bearing on the initial steps taken in response to overuse pain (you'll want to modify your training and treat the inflammation no matter what's causing it), it is a vital measure in relation to treating the underlying cause and making sure it never returns. For this reason, you'll want to investigate the underlying cause even if the affected area responds quickly to the initial treatments.

Some overuse injuries are caused by poor technique, inappropriate equipment, or increasing training volume too rapidly. But most overuse injuries involve a muscular imbalance of some form. While there's generally no harm in assuming you have the imbalances most commonly associated with your condition and taking the corresponding corrective measures, the safest thing to do is visit a good physical therapist or chiropractor who understands swimming, cycling, and running biomechanics. A thorough examination from such an individual takes all the guesswork out of the diagnosis and subsequent rehabilitation.

4. Manage the Problem

When it comes to addressing the underlying cause of your overuse injury, the two measures you can take are those that manage the problem, and those that actually correct the problem. The latter are always preferable, of course, but they take time. Management measures can buy you that time. For example, overpronation of the foot during running can cause a few different overuse injuries. Installing corrective orthotics in your running shoes can effectively manage overpronation and get you back on the road while you make efforts to correct the abnormality that is the actual cause of the overpronation.

5. Correct the Problem

Your ultimate goal with respect to any overuse injury is not just to make it go away but also to keep it from ever coming back. This often entails correcting biomechanics and muscle imbalances. As I explained above, the way to correct muscle imbalances is to perform appropriate stretching and strengthening exercises on a consistent basis. This is also the first step in correcting technique, because muscle imbalances are often part of the cause of poor technique. But it is only the first step.

The next step is to have an expert (such as a coach or physical therapist) observe and suggest modifications to your technique, so that you get a sense of what proper technique feels and looks like. Then, using this information, begin to practice kinesthetic awareness—that is, pay attention to your technique during workouts and perform technique drills such as those described in the chapters on swim, bike, and run training. This process requires discipline and patience, because long-held habits of posture and movement are not changed in a day, but your discipline and patience will be rewarded, I promise.

Eight Common Overuse Injuries

Following are descriptions of the eight most common overuse injuries in triathlon, their symptoms, typical causes, and suggested treatments:

Swimmer's Shoulder

Swimmer's shoulder involves damage to the tendons and bursa deep inside the shoulder joint caused by impingement (pinching) during the freestyle arm stroke. The primary symptom is pain in this area, felt initially after swimming, and also during swimming in more advanced cases.

Factors that frequently contribute to swimmer's shoulder include excessive or sudden increases in training volume, technique flaws, and muscular imbalances. All three factors are interdependent. Technique flaws lead to muscle imbalances, muscle imbalances exacerbate technique flaws, and swimming in a fatigued state (as one does more frequently at higher training volumes) worsens both. The technique flaws most commonly associated with swimmer's shoulder are failure to maintain a high elbow during the recovery phase and crossing the midline during the pull phase of the arm cycle. The muscle imbalances associated with swimmer's shoulder are tightness in the chest and shoulder deltoids and weakness in the rotator cuff muscles and the shoulder stabilizers in the upper back.

Exercises like the Two Arm Twist are effective means of correcting these causal imbalances, especially when combined with kinesthetic awareness and technique alteration in the pool. Doing these exercises will strengthen your core muscles and your shoulder girdle and will teach your body to dissociate hip movements from back movements. You will be able to feel these effects while swimming, and they can provide a platform for kinesthetic awareness and technique modifications, which will not come as easily without such a platform. A short-term reduction in swimming volume is almost always required in cases of swimmer's shoulder, both to allow healing and to lessen the amount of swimming you do in a fatigued state.

Lower Back Pain

A fair number of runners and swimmers experience lower back pain, but it's best known as a cyclist's injury. The reason for the commonality of lower back pain in cyclists is the extremely crouched posture associated with cycling. The spinal erector muscles become progressively overstretched until micro-tears occur, and with them the onset of pain.

In many cases, improving bike setup can mitigate lower back pain. However, in order to resolve it completely and prevent its return, you'll most likely need to strengthen the muscles of your lower abdomen and lower back using exercises such as the Forward Roll.

Runner's Knee

Runner's knee is the common name for chondromalacia, an overuse condition wherein the cartilage underneath the kneecap begins to wear due to friction caused by improper tracking of the kneecap during the running motion. The noticeable symptoms are inflammation and pain under the kneecap during running.

The main biomechanical factors associated with runner's knee are overpronation of the foot and imbalance between the quadriceps and hamstrings (that is, relatively weak and loose quadriceps and relatively tight hamstrings). The latter condition can cause the kneecap to track improperly and can also cause or exacerbate overpronation.

Two management devices, shoe orthotics and knee straps, can be effective in helping athletes continue running while they work to correct the imbalances that are causing the kneecap to track improperly. Since so many different biomechanical factors are potential culprits in cases of runner's knee, it can be helpful to have your stride analyzed by an expert, who can identify the abnormalities that are probably contributing to your problem. Or you can simply perform the stretching and strengthening routines I've described, which are designed to correct the imbalances that are most common in triathletes, and then seek stride analysis only if these programs don't seem to help your condition.

Hamstring Strain

Hamstring strains are partial or complete tears in groups of muscle fibers in one or more of the three hamstring muscles. They occur most often near tendons at the top (near the butt) or bottom (near the knee) of the muscle. Hamstring strains can be acute (sudden) or chronic, developing slowly over time. The former are more common in sports that involve sprinting. Chronic strains are more common among distance runners and triathletes. As the tears that constitute muscle strains happen literally through overstretching, tightness of the hamstring muscles is regarded as the most common contributor to this form of injury. However, some researchers have noted that relative weakness of the hamstrings also correlates with hamstring strains. Weak lower abdominals and glutes and tight hip flexors are commonly seen in hamstring strain sufferers.

Hamstring strains can linger for a very long time and recur with maddening frequency, so you should address symptoms and their underlying causes swiftly and aggressively. Rest if necessary, and as long as necessary, and use icing, anti-inflammatories, massage, and compression bandaging liberally. Do longer and more gradual warm-ups, as failure to warm up properly may be a contributing cause of hamstring strains. Performing functional strengthening exercises for the hamstrings will increase muscle fiber recruitment during running and thereby lessen the stress placed on individual fibers.

Iliotibial Band Syndrome

The iliotibial band (or IT band) is the largest tendon in the body, running from above the hip joint on the back side of the body to below the knee joint on the frontal shin. Studies of the running biomechanics of runners with IT band syndrome have revealed that it is caused by rubbing of the band against the bone during one brief segment of the striding motion. At high training volumes, this constant rubbing causes inflammation. The noticeable symptom of IT band syndrome is pain centralized above and outside the knee or just below the hip socket.

In most cases, the proximate cause of IT band syndrome is weak hip abductors (muscles on the outside of the thigh). When these muscles are weak, the pelvis tilts to the side when one foot is planted and the other foot is elevated, causing overstretching and rubbing of the IT band on the planted leg. The Multidirectional Lunge exercise described above is an excellent functional strengthener of the hip abductors. Sports massage is a helpful management device, as it loosens the band and thereby lessens the amount of friction that occurs during running.

Shin Splints

Doctors are not yet certain exactly what shin splints are, physiologically, but runners and triathletes know that, experientially, a shin splint is a pain on the medial (inside) or front of the shin that occurs during running. Such pains result from increasing running mileage too quickly. The medial variety is most common. Shin splints nearly always occur in just one leg at a time—specifically, the runner's dominant leg.

Medial shin splints are associated with imbalances in the muscles of the lower leg, while anterior shin splints are associated with overpronation. Treat shin splints by reducing running volume or ceasing to run entirely, reducing the inflammation, stretching the calf muscles frequently, and performing the corrective exercises for the lower leg described earlier.

Achilles Tendinitis

Achilles tendinitis is inflammation of the Achilles tendon, which connects the two major muscles of the calf, the gastrocnemius and the soleus, to the heel bone. In severe cases, the tendon can develop nodules of scar tissue or even rupture. The most common causes of Achilles tendinitis are tight calf muscles and overpronation of the foot.

When symptoms appear, take all the usual measures to reduce inflammation. If overpronation is a factor, switch to more stable shoes or get orthotics to manage the problem in the short term. Stretch your calf muscles frequently and strengthen their antagonists using corrective exercises for the lower leg. Work to undo any other imbalances that may be contributing to your overpronation.

Plantar Fasciitis

The plantar fascia is a tough band of tissue that originates in the heel and spreads like a web toward the forefoot. Its main job is to maintain the arch through the gait motion (walking or running). Plantar fasciitis involves tearing and scarring of the plantar fascia, usually near the heel bone, that occurs due to overstretching of the fascia during the foot strike portion of the running stride. The classic early symptom of plantar fasciitis is pain felt deep in the heel when walking first thing in the morning and when beginning to run. As the condition worsens, pain will last longer in the morning and during workouts. Untreated, plantar fasciitis can become so painful that running is impossible.

The common muscular and biomechanical problems associated with plantar fasciitis are overpronation of the foot, a high, inflexible arch, and imbalance in the muscles of the lower leg. Address lower leg muscle imbalances with frequent stretching of the calves and the Achilles tendon and with exercises that strengthen the medial and frontal shin muscles. Wearing a tension night splint will help the fascia heal at a functional length. Wearing boots or high heels helps by giving the fascia a break from the usual flex and pressure.

Preventing and Dealing with Illness and General Fatigue

You can do more than you might think to prevent general fatigue—a great epidemic in our society to which triathletes are especially susceptible—and the viral infections associated with colds and flu. The various measures you can take fall into four categories: diet, sleep, stress reduction, and foiling germs. Let's take a look at each of them.

Diet

Nutrition supports every physical process from breathing to thought. You can do literally nothing without it. The immune system, too, is deeply dependent on dietary nutrients, including antioxidant vitamins such as C and E, and minerals such as zinc. As much as possible, obtain these vitamins and minerals from natural foods, as these contain phytochemicals that also support immunity and are not to be found in dietary supplements. Note that there's no conclusive evidence that popular herbs such as Echinacea and green tea make a difference in the prevention or treatment of infection.

Vigorous endurance workouts result in the release of stress hormones such as cortisol that suppress the immune system and leave athletes susceptible to viral infection for many hours after the workout is completed. For this reason, serious endurance athletes get colds and flus about as often as sedentary people, whereas those who exercise moderately get fewer. However, research has shown that consuming carbohydrate during and after exercise (most likely in the form of a sports drink) can blunt the release of stress hormones and their weakening effect on the immune system.

Sleep

Sleep deprivation is more or less an illness in itself and it also increases one's susceptibility to contracting other illnesses such as colds and flu.

Of particular interest to triathletes are sleep's effects on glucose metabolism and production of the hormones cortisol and human growth hormone (HGH). Lack of sufficient sleep reduces the body's ability to process glucose, and therefore to produce energy. It also heightens levels of cortisol, which attacks muscle tissue and must be suppressed in order for proper post-workout tissue repair to occur. What's more, HGH, the anabolic (i.e., muscle-building) hormone that plays the biggest role in rebuilding tissue after exercise, requires sleep for full activation, so the less sleep you get, the less usable muscle you wake up with. Sleep loss also reduces the activity of interleukins, a group of molecules involved in signaling between cells of the immune system.

All of this is bad news for many triathletes, because chronic sleep deprivation is a bona fide epidemic in Western society. The average adult sleeps 90 minutes less today than a century ago. A majority of Americans now sleep less than eight hours a night, which is the very *minimum* that most people need, according to sleep experts. Whatever you're staying awake for, it can't be worth more than your health. Go to bed. Get those extra 30 or 60 minutes of shut-eye, either at night or in the form of a nap, and watch your performance and all-around vitality take off.

Stress Reduction

From a biological perspective, stress is not feeling tense or frazzled. Rather, it's any activity or experience that taxes the body in a way that requires the release of certain hormones, especially adrenaline. The list of activities and experiences that fit this description is very long. In fact, it's not misleading to say that the more you do in a day—regardless of what you do—the more stress your body endures. Overworked adrenal glands are a common symptom of the stress that is so prevalent in our society. If you feel run-down fairly often, chances are good that your adrenal glands are overworked and that you're doing too much in life. It's hard to swim against the current of society; it would be extremely facile of me to blithely advise you simply to "do less." Nevertheless, you need to be aware of these facts, and I'm confident that such awareness can lead eventually to meaningful changes in how you manage your life.

Stress is also a potent suppressor of the immune system. Whether psychological or physical in origin, stress causes the release of the hormones cortisol and adrenaline in the body. These hormones inhibit the production of T cells, which are special white blood cells whose job is to locate and destroy antigens ("foreign invaders" in the body). One clinical study showed that the presence of stress can double one's risk of contracting a cold.

Stressors do not affect everyone the same way. Some of us are high reactors, meaning we have a strong physiological response to stressors, while others are low reactors. All of us, high reactors especially (and I believe that a disproportionate number of triathletes are high reactors), need to learn to treat stress as the killer it is. Heighten your awareness of its symptoms, some of which are very subtle, and maintain a vigilant lookout for them. Condition yourself to avoid its avoidable causes and make it a point to experience the relaxation response that is its antidote on a daily basis. Exercise is among the best relaxation techniques around, but if approached in the wrong frame of mind it, too, can become a stressor.

Foiling Germs

Colds and flus occur when viral bacteria make a home inside your body. There are some effective prophylactic means of foiling these germs' plans of corporeal takeover. One is simply to avoid high-risk environments, which can be defined as large numbers of people in closed spaces during the winter.

Another useful measure is the practice of germ hygiene. Most people think airborne germs are the leading cause of infection. Actually, it's self-inoculation, as when you grab a germ-infested doorknob and then slyly pick your nose with the same hand. The good news is that self-inoculation is largely avoidable: Just keep your hands away from your nose and eyes, and wash them frequently.

Flu shots are the simplest of all ways you can foil germs. Here's an immunity boost you can quantify: Flu vaccinations are 85 percent effective, and even when they're not, they tend to reduce the severity of infections. Once recommended only for the weak and elderly, they're now advised for all. October is the month to get one.

When you do get sick, you have two interrelated objectives: recovering quickly and minimizing lost training time. Research has shown that exercising with cold symptoms is not a problem. Head colds generally do not hamper exercise performance significantly and exercise does not increase the duration or severity of colds. When symptoms move into your chest and lungs, be cautious. Take a precautionary day off and follow up with a test workout the next day. If you feel bad, pull the proverbial ripcord. When you have flu symptoms such as fever and body aches, do not exercise at all, and do not resume exercise until a day or two after the symptoms have vanished.

Overtraining Syndrome

Overtraining syndrome denotes a decrease in performance capacity and other symptoms resulting from chronic failure to achieve adequate recovery or from maintaining a training workload that is beyond the athlete's absorption capacity for a long period of time. Often a loss of morale for training is part of the mix as well. The first observed symptom of overtraining is usually an unexpected leveling off and subsequent diminishment of performance. One or more of a long list of additional symptoms may also appear. These include insomnia, irritability, chronic fatigue, loss of appetite, headaches, weight loss, and nausea. In most cases, a drastic and lengthy reduction in training must occur before the athlete can begin to regain fitness.

Overtraining syndrome is rare except among athletes of a very high level of conditioning, because only such athletes can work too much and/or rest too little long enough for overtraining syndrome to result. The average triathlete does not experience overtraining syndrome but simply overtrains. In other words, the average triathlete cannot work too much or rest too little for more than a week or two without incurring an injury or seeing a drop in performance, and this drop will not be the irreversible tailspin associated with overtraining syndrome but only a minor setback that can be resolved with a few days of rest and light training.

It's easy enough to prevent overtraining syndrome. The most effective objective early warning device is monitoring your morning heart rate. Your morning heart rate should gradually decrease or hold steady throughout the training cycle. Any increase is a potential sign of incomplete recovery. A single high measurement is nothing to worry about, but an upward *trend* is always a bad sign that you should address immediately. You can also catch early symptoms of overtraining through subjective self-observation. Never should a full week go by without your having at least one good workout, which is to say, a workout in which you feel very good in relation to the specific task you're performing and your present level of fitness. Generally, you'll want to have far more than one good workout each week, of course, but what I'm trying to say is that you should not let more than one bad week pass before you modify your training to correct your work-recovery ratio. Nip it in the bud, as they say.

Your Triathlon Staff

*I*magine what it would be like to live and train at the U.S. Olympic Training Center in Colorado Springs as a member of the USA Triathlon Resident Teams. You'd receive daily personal coaching from one of the best coaches in the sport, plus supplemental coaching from worthy assistants. Men and women in white coats would subject you to physiological testing, the results of which would be used to chart the most appropriate course for your training. You'd get a free weekly sports massage and access to physical therapists when you needed them. All your meals would be cooked for you.

Well, you're not a member of the Resident Teams, but that doesn't mean you can't duplicate the advantages of USOTC residency wherever you happen to be. I like to encourage triathletes to conceive of themselves as having their own support staff. Thinking in this way will help you take the fullest advantage of the professionals of various kinds whose services can improve your bottom line as a triathlete.

As a minimum, your support staff should include your primary care physician, the staff of the stores where you do your multisport shopping, and probably a group swim coach. Triathletes should choose their doctors with triathlon in mind. Relatively few doctors know how to handle athletes. I've had doctors who did not even touch the injury with which I came to them. You don't want that. You want the kind of doctor who takes athletes seriously, views complete rest as a last resort, and who has a network of athlete-oriented physical therapists, massage therapists, and other professionals to whom he or she will refer you when necessary.

Select your gear and equipment retailers, and especially your bike shop, with equal care. The stores whose personnel are true experts in bike fitting and who take real care with repairs and tune-ups are in the minority, and they make a big difference.

Your support staff can also include a running coach, a cycling coach, a triathlon coach, a nutritionist, a massage therapist, a sports psychologist, a chiropractor, an acupuncturist, and/or a personal trainer. High-quality professionals in each of these categories can have a profound impact on your fitness and racing, and perhaps even on your enjoyment of the sport. You probably don't need all of them—at least not all at once—but it doesn't hurt to consider each as an option. If you stay open to various possibilities, you can get the help you need when you need it without wasting a lot of time running from expert to expert or spending a lot of money on each. For example, you might find an employee at your local health foods market who's an endurance athlete himself and knows a lot about nutrition. You might get your sports psychology from a book and your triathlon coaching through one of the Internet-based coaching services that now exist. A number of triathletes in my area participate in group run workouts led by a terrific running coach who has run a 2:13 marathon and trained several Olympians. They pay $20 a month for his services. Such possibilities do exist!

The lone nonprofessional member of your support staff will probably be your spouse or significant other—the one person who's actually willing to rise with you at 4:45 A.M. on a Sunday morning, help you with the logistics of getting ready to race, and yell encouragement during your race. While this person is, of course, much more to you than a member of your triathlon support crew, this fact itself can be the very thing that makes him or her the most valuable member of your crew. Hearing my name shouted in the unmistakable timbre of my wife's voice gives me a greater energy boost than anything I might swallow from a water bottle or gel pack.

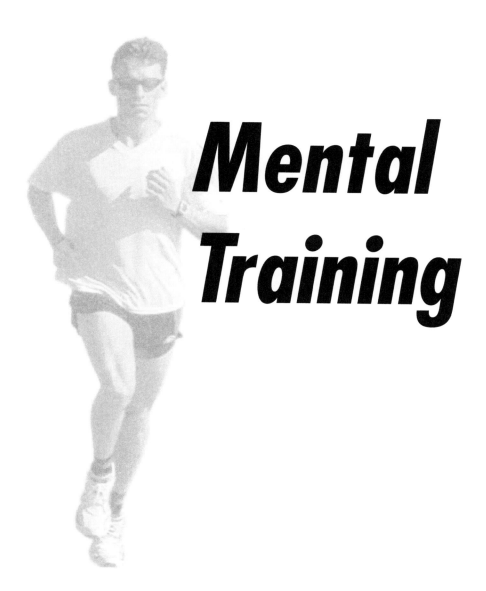

CHAPTER 9

Mental Training

I once asked six-time Hawaii Ironman winner Dave Scott to predict how triathlon training might evolve in the future, and with nary a pause he replied, "There's no question, the component of triathlon training that is lagging behind the rest is the mental component. I think we haven't done a very good job of integrating psychology into training programs. A few triathletes do a very good job of it, but most of us do not. We give it a lot of lip service, and that's about all."

There are probably a few reasons why this is so, but the main one would seem to be the traditional Western division of mind and body. Because we tend to think of the mind and the body as separate, and because on the surface sports appear to be a body thing, we focus on training the body for competition and more or less ignore the mind, or, if we don't ignore the mind, we certainly do not train it in the systematic way that we train the body. I believe it's not only possible but essential that you train your mind as consciously and programmatically as you train your body if you wish to make progress as a triathlete. *Real* mental training entails cultivating certain mental skills that are beneficial to triathletes, practicing a variety of effective mental techniques within and between workouts, and implementing proven strategies for dealing with the various challenges triathletes normally face.

Mental Skills

Triathlon performance depends on a variety of physical skills, or attributes, ranging from strong lungs to good swim technique. But it does not depend on these alone. Triathlon performance is also supported by mental skills, which are the psychological attributes that help you make the most of the physical skills you develop in training. There are seven primary mental skills that serve the triathlete: motivation, playfulness, determination, discipline, confidence, optimism, and mindfulness. Let's take a close look at each of these skills, and how to nurture them.

Motivation

Triathlon is voluntary. Training begins with a motivation to train, and racing, with a desire to compete. Without such self-generated urges, training and racing do not happen. A motivation is simply a felt reason, or set of reasons, to act. Put another way, it is a sense of there being a clear personal benefit in taking some action. Among triathletes, the following motivations to train and compete are most common: enjoyment of the activities of swimming, cycling, and running; improvement or hope for improvement; fitness and health; camaraderie; victory (either relative or absolute); reputation and vanity.

None of these motivations is inherently better or worse than any other. However, there is one that no triathlete can do without: enjoyment of the activities themselves. The rest are gravy, as they say. For when it comes to motivation, the one rule is this: Get it where you can, because the more motivated you are toward your pursuit of triathlon, the more success and fulfillment you'll achieve in it. Motivation is not an all-or-nothing affair. It has infinite degrees. If you have no motivation for triathlon, you should quit the sport. There's no shame in it. But as long as you have some motivation, you may as well have a lot.

Each person is motivated in his or her own way, and most people have different motivations at different times. Consider your own motivations as a triathlete and nourish them as much as you can. For example, if you are strongly motivated by camaraderie, give yourself every opportunity to train in groups. Or if you are strongly motivated by victory, set results-related goals, learn the name of the person in your age group who just barely beat you last time and try to beat him or her next time.

But always keep it in mind that the one essential motivator is enjoyment of the activities of swimming, cycling, and running themselves, and let nothing get in the way of this. By enjoyment I mean something very specific—namely, the good feeling that is associated with being totally absorbed in some challenge, as when a child plays, a painter paints, a surgeon operates, or an athlete competes in "the zone." We enjoy activities when they require us to utilize the full potential of certain abilities we possess. This kind of situation requires a suspension of self-consciousness that leads to our in a sense *becoming* the activities we pursue, which, for whatever reason, feels very good.

Through exhaustive research, the psychologist Mihaly Csikszentmihalyi was able to demonstrate that people in all walks of life, from every culture, and of all ages and both genders experience enjoyment in the same general way and in the same general kinds of situations. According to Csikszentmihalyi, the types of situation that best facilitate enjoyment (which he calls "flow") have the following characteristics: 1) they are well-defined tasks with clear definitions of success and failure; 2) they facilitate concentration; 3) the participant brings a goal to them; 4) they offer clear feedback regarding progress toward the goal; 5) the participant is able to be totally unselfconscious in them; 6) the participant has a feeling of sufficient but not absolute control vis-à-vis the outcome of the task; and 7) participation in the task is likely to yield improvement in the skills involved.

As you can see, triathlon training and competition have the potential to fulfill these conditions perfectly. But it's not automatic. Various factors, including self-doubt and lack of (appropriate) goals, can stand in the way of your becoming completely absorbed in the training or racing experience and thereby deprive you of your most important motivator. It is essential that you never lose sight of the importance of enjoyment and keep a watchful eye on factors that could spoil it.

Playfulness

Triathlon is a form of play. It is a sport, after all, and a hobby, and sports and hobbies are played. Playfulness is simply the attitude with which one approaches play. To have a playful attitude toward triathlon does not mean we fail to take it seriously, but only that we refuse to take it too seriously. This attitude is indispensable to the triathlete, because it is a fundamental condition of enjoyment. When you take a sport or hobby too seriously, you don't allow yourself to enjoy it *unless you obtain specific results from it*. This not only leaves your happiness too much to chance, but it is actually a surefire way to obtain worse results than you would with a more relaxed perspective. It is human nature to give a better effort when you're loose and having fun than when you're uptight and edgy. I'm not sure why this is so, but it clearly is the case. As the former world champion marathoner Ian Thompson said, "When I am happy I am running well, and when I am running well I am happy."

Competitive triathletes commit the error of staking their happiness on specific results all too frequently. For example, American Siri Lindley was once strongly favored to earn a position on the 2000 U.S. Olympic Triathlon Team. However, she psyched herself out by placing too much pressure on herself to fulfill this expectation and wound up racing poorly in the Olympic Trials. This devastating disappointment inspired Lindley to get her priorities straight and turn her focus back on enjoying herself, come what may. One year after missing out on the Olympics, and racing with a new attitude, she won the Triathlon World Championship. The moral could not be plainer. Always approach triathlon with a playful attitude. If you do, you'll have more fun and better results—maybe not a world championship title in your case, but worthy results nonetheless!

Determination

As a triathlete, you need determination in order to overcome suffering and give all you have when racing. This determination comes from within you, but it is released by nothing more or less than a sense of the meaningfulness of the race itself. Contrary to popular assumption, determination is not something that some people have and others do not. All of us have determination with respect to the things that matter most to us. When a goal is sufficiently meaningful for you, you *will* show determination in pursuing it. When it lacks sufficient meaningfulness, you will not be able to give a total effort to achieve it.

There are a couple of ways you can increase your determination to overcome suffering in races. First, you can actively build up the importance of individual triathlons in your mind for the sake of releasing your determination within them. You can make individual triathlons more meaningful to you by designating a small number of chosen triathlons (one to three a year) as peak races, by setting challenging goals for these events, and by beginning to prepare for them long in advance of their happening. However, while heaping anticipation on these events, just be sure never to stake your happiness on achieving certain results in them, or you'll psych yourself out. Focus on giving your best effort.

A second way to increase your determination is to stake your self-image on your ability to overcome suffering—that is, to make determination itself more important to you—by engaging in a certain kind of self-talk during races. "If I don't push through this, I'll know I'm a wimp, and I'll never let myself live it down." That kind of thing. I began using this tactic in every race after I finished a few triathlons knowing that I'd held back just a bit for fear of suffering. I decided that the shame I felt when I did not show true determination was more unbearable than the suffering associated with showing true determination, and I began to act accordingly. It worked. One caution: Sometimes it's just not your day and you really are better off pulling back or throwing in the towel.

Even great athletes struggle with determination. After winning his second Hawaii Ironman World Championship, Canadian Peter Reid had a series of disastrous races, finishing only one triathlon in the next 18 months. Following yet another DNF in Australia, a frustrated Reid, threatening retirement, admitted to the press that he had suffered so greatly in that second Ironman victory, he was just plain afraid to race that hard again, hence his loss of determination. Happily, by at last confronting the problem squarely, he was able to overcome it and return to form.

In most cases, the more often you push through suffering, the more natural (I won't say "the easier") it becomes to do it again. All forms of suffering become less acute as they become more familiar. Herein lies a third means of maximizing your determination in triathlon. When suffering, think about past times when you've suffered greatly and pushed through it, and how proud you felt afterward.

Discipline

If determination is significant mostly in relation to racing, discipline is significant mostly in relation to training. Discipline in training is a matter of having a plan and sticking to it. There are really two sides to this attribute, however: initiative, on the one hand, and restraint, on the other. Initiative is the discipline to do enough, while restraint is the discipline not to do too much. Some triathletes have no trouble motivating themselves to work out every day, but have a difficult time holding back when they should. It takes discipline, for example, to cut back on one's training sufficiently during a taper period, to silence one's irrational fear that tapering will result in the loss of fitness. Other triathletes find it more challenging to train consistently or plan ahead.

Few triathletes are strong in both initiative and restraint. You must practice both kinds of discipline in your training in order to realize your full potential. One effective way to find the right balance between the two is by training with a partner who is strong where you are weak. Another way is to find a good coach. As an athlete, I find that an outside perspective, even when not technically an expert perspective, often makes up for blind spots in my own perspective and keeps me from going off track (always in the direction of lack of restraint).

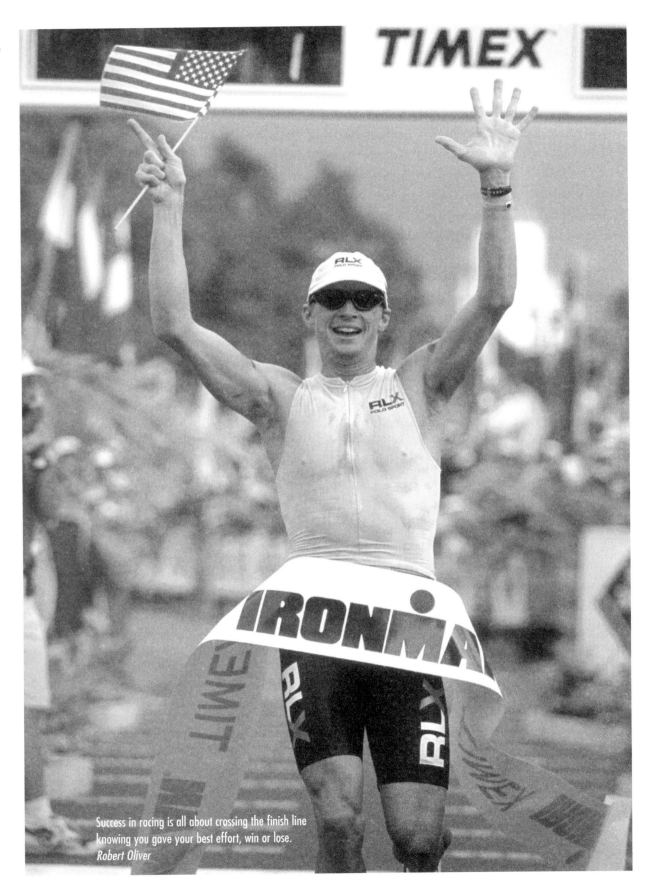

Success in racing is all about crossing the finish line
knowing you gave your best effort, win or lose.
Robert Oliver

Confidence

Confidence has to do with believing you can do what you want to do. True confidence is not wishful thinking but rather a rational expectation of success that is based in experience and an accurate knowledge of one's abilities. As such, true confidence can only be increased through success. Yet success happens all the time. Every good workout is a success, as are each period of consistent training and every lesson learned.

But there is such a thing as overconfidence. An athlete becomes overconfident when his or her sense of what is possible becomes detached from reality. This is generally self-correcting: The overconfident athlete falls far short of expectations and learns to generate more reasonable expectations for the next challenge. However, some athletes have a habit of chronic excuse making that allows them to consistently maintain an inflated view of their abilities. Usually, such athletes maintain this view mostly for the sake of impressing others with it, and thus it is a character flaw. Don't be this person.

The triathletes who have the most *true* confidence are those who make the most of the successes they've experienced. They *know* they can achieve the goals they set for themselves and refuse to lose faith until and unless they come up short in the end. When they race and find themselves struggling to achieve a goal, they think about their best workouts and races, which *prove* they can do what they're trying to do, not about their inner doubts. I've done my share of post-race interviews with champion triathletes, and over and over again I've heard these men and women say, in explaining their victory, "I just had confidence in my training (or fitness)." Successful triathletes actively use their confidence to conquer challenges when racing. You can easily do the same. In training, practice calling to mind your best moments frequently, as a matter of habit, and your confidence will grow and eventually serve you well in competition.

Optimism

Like confidence, optimism has to do with believing in success, but unlike confidence, optimism is a general disposition that's detached from experience and fact and applies equally to all desired outcomes. As such, optimism is not unlike overconfidence, except that overconfidence is an overestimation of one's own abilities, whereas optimism is an outward-looking sense of hope and possibility. Optimists tend to simply *expect* success regardless of whether they have legitimate reasons to do so. The psychologist Martin Seligman demonstrated through a career's worth of experimentation that optimism plays as significant a role in success in all undertakings, including sport, as talent and determination. However, one's overall disposition toward optimism or pessimism forms in early childhood, so becoming fundamentally more optimistic as an adult requires an investment of time and effort.

The hallmark of pessimism is fatalism, or becoming easily discouraged. To train yourself to become more optimistic, first start paying attention to how you deal with setbacks. When you catch yourself saying things like "Here we go again!" or "I *knew* this would happen!" *dispute* these words of discouragement. Don't let yourself expect the worst or give up too quickly, as pessimistic beliefs have a way of being self-fulfilling. Over time, if you're vigilant in this manner, you can train yourself to expect the best, which also has a way of being self-fulfilling.

Mindfulness

In relation to sport, mindfulness is the capacity to make use of information that is relevant to performance. In triathlon, mindfulness can help you do everything from improve your technique to figure out the race nutrition strategy that works best for you. Various forms of denial and inattention (the opposites of mindfulness) are among the primary causes of athletes' failure to achieve optimal performance. A good example is not paying attention to signs of general fatigue. Mindfulness is a necessary component of everything you do as a triathlete—there is not one aspect of your pursuit of triathlon that cannot get a boost from greater awareness.

The tricky thing about mindfulness is that it can be enhanced only through the willful practice of mindfulness—a classic catch-22. A good way to start is by getting into the habit of concentrating on your body while you work out. By doing this, you can't help but notice patterns that can prove useful. For example, during one recent track workout I noticed that I tend to squint my eyes when I grow fatigued while running at a high intensity level, and that by consciously relaxing my face I could keep my whole body more relaxed and actually feel the suffering less. This after 18 years of running.

Mental Training Techniques

When you're awake, you're thinking. There's no stopping this. You think throughout every workout and race, and you often think triathlon-related thoughts or other thoughts that affect your pursuit of triathlon even when you're not working out or racing. Thinking the right kinds of thoughts at such times can be very beneficial with respect to your pursuit of triathlon, especially when these thoughts are practiced consciously and formally as mental training techniques. I will here discuss six such techniques: setting goals, body awareness, self-talk, visualization, self-observation, and directed thinking.

Setting Goals

There are many helpful ways to set goals as a triathlete. They can be quantitative or qualitative, short-term or long-term, minor or major, and race-related or training-related. You should make use of each of these varieties of goal in your pursuit of triathlon. Goal setting is a very powerful way of enhancing your motivation to train and race and of improving performance.

Perhaps you've heard of the SMART acronym in relation to goal setting. It is said that appropriate goals are specific, measurable, attainable, relevant, and time-bound. Usually I find such acronyms hokey, but this one is right on the money. Unless a goal is specific, it is not really even a goal and you have no way of knowing whether or when you've achieved it. "I want to improve my weaknesses" is not a specific goal. "I want to improve my swim technique and my ability to run off the bike" is better. Similarly, it's difficult to observe progress toward a goal if it is not measurable in one way or another. Improvements in swim technique and in one's ability to run off the bike can be measured in time, but time is not the only way to measure triathlon goals. Appropriate goals are also neither easy nor impossible to attain. Remember, the real purpose of goals is to motivate progress, and people are motivated most when there's hope but not certainty. The goals you select also need to make sense in relation to the entire constellation of goals and desires you have as a triathlete. "I want to beat my training partner Tony in every workout" is probably not a relevant goal if being properly trained for races is also a goal. And lastly, a goal is also not a goal unless it has a due date attached to it. For example, "I want to improve my swim technique and my ability to run off the bike" would work well under the heading "Goals for Next Season."

You should set one or more measurable goals for each race. "I want to finish," "I want to break three hours," and "I want to place in my age group" are good examples of such goals (if they're indeed attainable). If you set an overall time goal, you may also wish to set swim, bike, and run split goals (and possibly even transition time goals) underneath it. Doing so can give you a better feeling for what it will take to achieve the overall goal. Setting a goal range or two tiers of goals is acceptable in some situations, as in "I'd like to break the world record, but I'll be satisfied with a course record." Modifying your goals (up or down) mid-race is also sometimes necessary or appropriate. Examples of worthy nonquantitative races goals are "not to panic during the swim start" and "to do a better job of keeping hydrated throughout the race."

It's a good practice to set seasonal goals when planning each upcoming season. These can include performance goals, areas of improvement goals, and measurable training goals. You should approach each week of training with the goal of successfully completing the training you've planned, and approach each of your long and quality workouts with specific performance goals in mind, as in "I'd like to complete my 35-mile long ride in two hours." The more goals the better, really, as long as each goal adheres to the principles I've outlined, and you never lose sight of the fact that failure to achieve any particular goal is not a failure in the truest sense if the goal has motivated you to give your best effort.

Body Awareness

As an athlete, you need to be able to read your body in a variety of ways. Pacing yourself during a race, improving your bike setup, knowing when to take a day off, keeping your form relaxed and correct despite fatigue, and a hundred other types of decisions you make and tasks you perform as a triathlete will all be made and performed more effectively with refined body awareness. Experience, more than anything, cultivates body awareness, but not all athletes make equal use of equal experience. In order to make the most of the experience you accumulate, you need to consciously ground yourself in your body during workouts, much as Zen practitioners do during meditation.

You feel a thousand different things while exercising. For example, you feel your left pinkie—but whether you actually notice how your left pinkie feels depends on whether you choose to focus your attention upon it. Practicing body awareness is a matter of focusing your attention sequentially on specific components of your overall experience, for the sake of assessing how you're doing and what you need and making decisions. You don't need to do this all the time while training, but you should do it more often and with more purpose than you would if you just allowed your mind to wander in every workout.

An important subspecies of body awareness that I've mentioned earlier is kinesthetic awareness, which is awareness of your body in space. Cultivating and making use of this awareness are crucial to developing proper biomechanics and technique in swimming, biking, and running. The whole bundle of sensations that comprise the experience of swimming, cycling, and running is infinitely more complex than one might assume as an observer. You can spend 40 years performing swim, bike, and run workouts and not stop noticing things you've never noticed before—things you can use—as long as you pay attention. For example, the great Lance Armstrong had already been a world-class cyclist for years before he evolved the high-cadence style of riding that made him a multiple Tour de France champion.

You should spend some time paying attention to all aspects of your body's movement in each of your workouts, devoting special attention to flaws you're trying to correct or technique elements you're trying to cultivate. For example, in a particular cycling workout you might choose to concentrate on your ankle action during the pedal stroke. Additionally, you should regularly perform technique drills in all three disciplines such as those described in earlier chapters and, of course, concentrate on your technique while you perform them.

Kinesthetic awareness is most effective when coupled with an outside perspective on your form, like that of a Masters swim coach, as it helps you know what you ought to be doing differently. Running on a treadmill and cycling on a wind trainer in view of a mirror can also reveal form flaws you never knew you had. Coupling kinesthetic awareness with corrective exercise is also highly beneficial, as muscle imbalances are a causal factor in relation to many form irregularities and corrective exercise makes your muscles better suited to proper form.

Self-Talk

Although it carries psycho-fluffy connotations, self-talk is something each of us does most of the time when training and racing. It's fundamental to the normal flow of consciousness. As a mental training technique, self-talk differs from spontaneous self-talk in that you take control of your inner chatter and give it a purpose. The logic behind the practice of this technique is simple: If you're going to talk to yourself anyway, you may as well say what you need to hear.

Like our conversations with others, our internal monologues tend to follow certain scripts. That is, we tend to think the same thoughts each time we encounter a particular type of situation in training and racing. Some of these thoughts are more helpful than others. Start paying attention to the things you tell yourself during challenging moments in training and racing and parse the effective messages ("I'm fit, I'm ready, I can do this") from ineffective ones ("I suck, I'm quitting"). Use your developing awareness to refine and improve the scripts you use, and use them consciously.

Visualization

After setting one of his many world records, the legendary Russian pole vaulter Sergei Bubka was asked by a reporter whether he had ever successfully cleared that height previously—in training, the reporter meant. "Yes, every night," Bubka replied, in reference to his nightly visualizations.

Most triathletes who practice visualization do so only in the few days or weeks before important races. This is better than nothing, but you really should practice visualization year-round, because, as the case of Bubka demonstrates so powerfully, visualization works. The body tends to move toward the mind's dominant thought. The more often you see yourself achieving your goals in your mind's eye, the more likely it is that you will eventually achieve these goals in reality.

At least once a week, find some quiet time, lie down, close your eyes, and imagine yourself racing successfully through all three legs of a triathlon. Try to make the vision as specific to your goals as possible. If your next big race is the Boonville Triathlon, let's say, then try to imagine yourself racing in Lake Boonville and on the streets of Boonville, and if your goal is to finish among the top 10 in your age group in this race, then imagine yourself doing precisely this.

Another way to visualize is with open eyes while you perform your swim, bike, and run workouts. That is, you can pretend you're racing while you're training. It's okay even to add an element of fantasy when practicing this form of visualization, for example by imagining yourself racing not for a top-10 age group finish in the Boonville Triathlon but for a gold medal in the Triathlon World Championship. While undeniably juvenile, such fantasizing provides the very serious benefit of generating excitement for racing, which will help you train harder and ultimately race better.

Self-Observation

Self-observation involves the same kind of internal scrutiny that's involved in the practice of body awareness, except that it takes a broader perspective in search of cause and effect. If all triathletes were the same, we could follow precisely the same training plans, diets, and so forth, and we wouldn't need self-observation. But each of us is a unique person with a unique life, and for this reason the practice of self-observation is crucial to our becoming better triathletes. View your development as a triathlete as an experiment of one, which is precisely what it is, and gather as much relevant data as you can find. That is, consistently pay close attention to how different eating patterns, training patterns, and equipment choices affect you, and use what you learn.

Pay attention also to your emotions as they relate to training and racing, because knowing your personality is as important to your athletic development as knowing your physical strengths and weaknesses. Discover what seems to motivate you, what spoils the fun, what increases your confidence, and so on. Use this information to lessen or eliminate unhelpful practices and influences from your training and your life, to maximize helpful ones, and to develop hypotheses that you can put to the test.

Directed Thinking

We humans are often slaves to our emotions, puppets to the strings of our brain chemistry. This tendency is bad not just from a mental health standpoint but also from an athletic standpoint, because if we cannot master our emotions, we cannot minimize negative emotions, which waste energy and cause us to perform beneath our true potential.

At the root, there is only one negative emotion: fear. The self-doubt that overtakes us just before the race starts, the urge to quit that gains sway when the race becomes painful, the brooding we do when we experience a setback in training—these emotions are all forms of fear, and all are counterproductive in relation to our desire to achieve success as triathletes. They are also perfectly natural emotions, however, and therefore impossible to eliminate. But we can contain them and in so doing minimize their impact.

The way to do so is through directed thinking. The term "directed thinking" was coined recently by a psychologist named A. B. Curtiss. The concept could not be simpler: Think what you want to think. Choose your thoughts. In particular, choose the thoughts that help—that make you relax when you're anxious, accepting when you're disappointed, and so forth. Rather than just allow yourself to feel fearful and think only thoughts suggested by your fears, separate your thoughts from your negative emotions through an act of will and give them a more constructive object.

For example, if you find yourself filled with self-doubt right before a race and suddenly second-guessing a goal you've considered perfectly reasonable for the past month, step away from this emotional state by labeling it as the natural manifestation of fear that it is, and then settle on a more productive thought, such as your recollection of having had this fear before and still gone out and achieved your original goal. Again, this technique will not often exterminate the negative emotion it combats, but it will prevent your being ruled by it, which will help you perform better in individual instances and make your overall life as a triathlete more pleasant in the aggregate.

One of the best uses I've made of directed thinking is turning *pain* into *effort* during workouts and races. It first happened spontaneously during a particular triathlon in which I felt mentally strong. Late in the bike segment, as the familiar burn and drain was coming on, it suddenly occurred to me that pain and effort are just two different perspectives on the same sensation, at least in the context of a test of endurance. But whereas pain is a helpless kind of feeling, a feeling of being the object of experiences, effort is a feeling of control, of *doing*. I found then, and I have found since then, that feeling effort is infinitely preferable to feeling suffering. It is more pleasant (or less unpleasant) and yields better results.

Mental Workouts

As you change clothes before a workout, you know more or less exactly what you're going to do with your body during the workout. You know how long the session will last, how it will be structured, how fast you'll go, and so forth. But every body workout is (or ought to be) a mental workout as well, and so you should begin it knowing what you'll do with your mind, too.

There are two general categories of mental approach to workouts that I recommend: one for high-intensity workouts and one for low-intensity workouts. During high-intensity workouts, you should practice the same set of mental techniques you would practice during a race, both because it will help you have a more successful workout and because it will give you more experience using these techniques. The most important technique to practice during hard workouts is body awareness. Concentrate your attention on the elements of your experience that keep your effort focused and your performance in line with your expectations. Monitor and control your pace, keep your breathing relaxed, keep your form efficient, etc. The other mental skill you should use in hard workouts is self-talk, to put yourself in the appropriate state of mental arousal right before the workout and to stay positive throughout the workout, especially toward the end. Use directed thinking as needed during these workouts.

For easier workouts, you can employ any of these same techniques and also visualization, but most often you should let your mind spin and go wherever it pleases. It may sound as though I'm saying the majority of your easier workouts should serve no mental purpose, but letting your mind spin serves a specific and highly valuable mental purpose:

relaxation. The spinning that your mind is able to do during workouts is one of the major reasons you complete them feeling calmed and refreshed. I wouldn't want to take that away from you!

Mental Challenges

The purpose of having the mental skills and techniques I've just talked about is to use them to overcome the mental challenges we face as triathletes. Among the most common and important mental challenges in triathlon are pre-race nerves, finding the zone in races, workout guilt, balancing triathlon and relationships, burnout, and training setbacks. Let's now discuss strategies for handling each of these challenges.

Pre-Race Nerves

Some athletes get so nervous before racing, they throw up. Others get only mild butterflies. Some begin feeling nervous weeks before the event takes place. Others remain calm until the final 24 hours. But every triathlete feels at least some nervousness in anticipation of racing.

Pre-race nerves are not intrinsically bad, but too much is unpleasant and can actually sabotage race performance. There's no single technique for dealing with pre-race nerves that works for every triathlete, but there are many techniques that work for some triathletes. The best general strategy to pursue by way of dealing with race nerves is to collect a few of these techniques that work for you and use them in combination. The techniques of directed thinking and self-talk that I discussed above are effective for lots of people. Use directed thinking to occupy your mind with whichever thought or other stimulus takes your mind furthest away from your squirming gut. Listening to music is one popular distraction. Use self-talk against what you believe to be the *source* of your nervousness, which for most triathletes is either fear of suffering or fear of failure or a mixture of the two. For example, to combat nervousness caused by fear of failure you might say to yourself, "Do the best you can." Repeat these messages over and over, as doing so not only strengthens the message but also channels nervous energy.

Some athletes find it helpful to perform a relaxation or breathing exercise prior to competing. For example, find a quiet place to sit, close your eyes, and simply inhale through your nose, exhale through your mouth, for a few minutes. Concentrate on your breathing and try to shut out all other thoughts and distractions.

Beyond these mental techniques that fight pre-race nerves by occu-

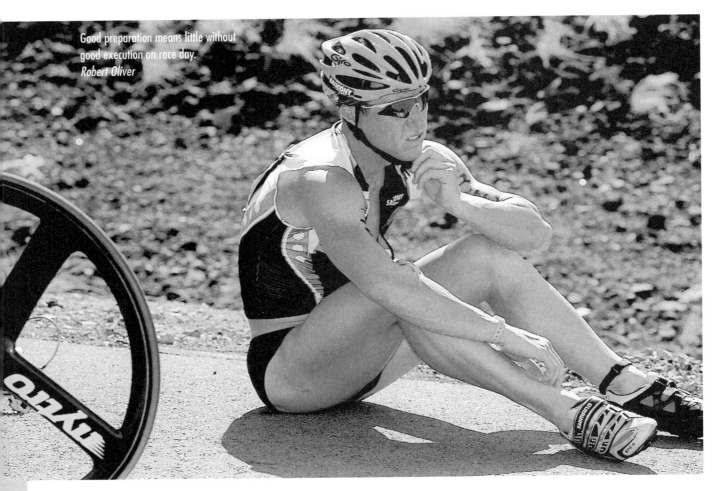

Good preparation means little without good execution on race day.
Robert Oliver

pying your mind, there are also ways to occupy your body that often work just as well. Their only limitation is that they only work on race morning. One such technique is to simply stay very busy between the time your alarm sounds and the time that starting horn sounds. Develop a race morning routine that keeps your mind and body focused on a series of tasks, not pointless tasks, but ones that you more or less must or should perform anyway. For that matter pointless activity, such as tossing a Yo-Yo or playing catch with a friend, can help as well.

Sports psychologists use the phrase "optimal arousal" (sounds kinky) to denote the emotional state that best prepares a particular athlete to perform well in a given sport. Optimal arousal is not the same for everyone. It depends on the personality. But optimal arousal tends to be similar for athletes in the same sport. For endurance athletes, optimal arousal is generally characterized by mild nervousness, moderate excitement, and focus. It's about halfway between where golfers want to be and where football players want to be prior to competing. Think about what constitutes your own optimal arousal state and about what you can do to achieve it before races.

Finding the Zone in Races

The so-called zone is that celebrated mental state wherein an athlete "becomes" the activity he or she is performing. It is a state of total concentration upon and absorption within the task at hand. This mental state is coveted not only because it is associated with peak performance but also because it is highly enjoyable. In endurance sports, especially, the zone is viewed as salvation because it allows one to master the prolonged discomfort that is an unavoidable part of the racing experience.

The zone is elusive, however. No triathlete has ever been able to find it in every race, and none ever will. But there are certain things you can do to maximize the chances of your finding the zone in any given race. I'll focus on two of them here. The first is timing your peak just right. When you've trained hard and intelligently and gotten all the rest you need, especially during the taper period, your body can be so ready to race that your mind has little choice but to follow along. Nothing puts you in the zone like feeling on. Have you ever noticed that how you feel in workouts has very little to do with how easy or hard you're working out and a lot to do with how strong your body feels in relation to what's being demanded of it? When you begin a workout in a fatigued or underprepared state, it doesn't matter how easy you go, you feel bad. When you begin a workout rested and well trained, it doesn't matter how hard you go, you feel good. Concentrate on getting your body in the zone for races, and your mind will get there, too.

On the strictly mental level, the most effective way to find the zone when racing is to concentrate on reading, interpreting, and using the many available sources of feedback. Try not to dissociate while racing—that is, hum tunes in your head or think about sex. Many triathletes do this naturally and genuinely feel that it helps; however, research has shown a powerful inverse relationship between the tendency to dissociate in competition and level of performance. In other words, winners think about the race. Remember, the definition of the zone is a state of total absorption in the task at hand. Such absorption is facilitated by your taking an all-business approach to racing, like a musician in recital, concentrating on any and all information that you need to make the operation a success. Look for split times and use them to monitor your pace. Pay attention to triathletes around you: Try to catch a competitor ahead of you, drop a competitor beside you, or draw energy from racing alongside a fellow triathlete. Take in fluids and other nutrition on a schedule. Keep your form relaxed and correct. Anticipate hills, aid stations, and so forth. Catalogue signs of pain and discomfort in your body and deal with each appropriately—this most often entails resisting general suffering. On a deeper level, immerse your

What to Think About (and What Not to Think About) During a Race

Do Think About:	Do Not Think About:
Your body: form, pace, effort, thirst, etc.	Your fears and doubts
Time: Monitor your pace, splits, progress, time remaining, etc.	Your suffering: Try to transform suffering into effort
Opponents: Draw energy from catching, staying ahead, or staying even with	Daydreams and distractions: Keep your mind on the race
Helpful thoughts: any positive message that helps you stay determined	
Your goals and strategy	

Table 9.1

mind in the sensations you experience while pushing forward against resistance. When you do a good job of keeping your mind focused on reading and using feedback while racing, you feel like the captain of a ship, in charge of your race, and that's a good feeling.

Workout Guilt

Workout guilt is the bane of the emotional life of many triathletes. By workout guilt I mean the gnawing, guilty feeling you experience when you miss one or more workouts, and sometimes even when you merely *think about* skipping a workout. Like other forms of guilt, workout guilt is not rational. It is a natural effect of emotional dependence on a habit. Ironically, those triathletes who train hardest (that is, who skip the fewest workouts) generally experience more workout guilt than those who train less, precisely because they are more emotionally dependent on the training habit.

A little workout guilt is not bad, but if you experience it often, something is wrong. Most often, frequent workout guilt is a sign that you've become too compulsive about training and need to lighten up. If you tend to dwell on a fear of losing fitness when you miss workouts, or if you go to extreme lengths to avoid missing workouts, you've simply lost touch with reality—in a way that's both common and understandable, but unhealthy nonetheless. Triathletes who do these things are more likely to be overtrained than undertrained. Very few triathletes, even among professionals, are able to be quite as consistent in their training as they would like to be. Distractions, setbacks, and changes in plan are all parts of the game. As long as your training schedule is generally manageable, there's no reason to panic about a missed workout here and there. If your training schedule is not manageable, that's a problem in itself. The fear of lost fitness is nearly always exaggerated. Research has shown that highly trained athletes who sharply reduce their training for a few days or even two weeks generally come back without missing a step.

Balancing Triathlon and Relationships

There is never enough time. And when you train for triathlons, time for other things, including important relationships, becomes even scarcer. Because it tends to entail a substantial time commitment, the pursuit of triathlon often causes triathletes' loved ones to feel neglected, a situation that inevitably leads to conflict and sometimes even to outright rupture, in cases of romantic partnerships. I've seen this happen several times, and it's no fun for either party.

As a married triathlete whose wife has zero interest in multisport, I am familiar with this challenge myself. But my wife and I have dealt with it pretty well, I think, so I can offer some advice you might be able to use in your own encounters with this classic situation. First, know that you have a right to be a triathlete. You may be married with several kids and a full-time job, but while these facts might make it difficult for you to be a triathlete, they do not make it wrong. Every person needs a hobby, something that's just for oneself, to say nothing of the need for exercise. Your spouse and/or other loved ones need to respect these rights and needs. Ask this person to kindly verbally confirm his or her understanding of the validity of your choice to be a triathlete.

But, of course, at the same time, you must respect your loved ones' need to spend time with you, which is also something you need. If you find yourself giving up this time all too easily, you're either in a relationship you should not be in or you've got your priorities scrambled. In either case, you must be fair, and you must not mistreat anyone who cares about you. It's a beautiful thing to have people in your life who want your time. Never take it for granted!

As with all relationship conflicts, the keys to mastering the triathlon time strain issue are communication and compromise. If your partner begins to show signs of resenting your devotion to triathlon, make an immediate effort to draw him or her into an honest, straightforward, and solution-oriented conversation, or series of conversations, about the issue. The strain can only worsen if you continue to communicate about it obliquely. The worst thing you can do is ignore or dismiss your partner's feelings. The next worst thing is to respond to indirect communication in kind.

Rarely, if ever, is this kind of situation resolved by one person's giving in completely. Some form of compromise is almost always required. Your insistence on having the freedom to enjoy the triathlon lifestyle is fair, while your mate's feeling of neglect is not unfounded. Compromising does not mean you have to do only half the amount of training needed to achieve an optimal performance. You might instead continue to train just as much, but find creative ways to include your family in some of your workouts, for example by letting your kids run around a soccer field while you circle the track that surrounds it. Another sort of compromise that often works is to ask for and receive permission to go ahead and neglect your family (to a degree) for a designated period of time while you train for the race of your life, after completing which you fully reimmerse yourself in family life forevermore. Be creative in your compromises. It's worth the effort.

Burnout

Every triathlete suffers the occasional period of burnout, or low motivation. Sometimes it lasts just a day or two, other times it is more protracted. Sometimes it's just a mild feeling of staleness or restiveness, other times a complete loss of desire to continue in the sport, even an aversion for it. Always there is a way to handle the particular form of burnout you're experiencing that will make things turn out for the best.

There are three basic ways to deal with feeling unmotivated for a particular workout. The first is just to suck it up and do the workout, knowing that you remain highly motivated toward the sport in general but are just having one of those days. Often, forcing yourself to work out when you don't feel like it provides a nice morale boost by demonstrating your discipline and willpower. A second way of dealing with a lapse of motivation is to let yourself off the hook and cancel the workout, guilt-free. This is generally the better solution when both your mind and your body could use the rest. A third type of solution entails tricking yourself into greater motivation by changing something about the planned workout. Instead of doing it alone, you can do it with a partner or group; instead of going hard, you can go easy; instead of riding on the road, you can pull out your mountain bike and ride off-road; whatever. You can even try buying yourself something new to use in or wear for the workout.

When a period of burnout lasts longer than a day or two and despite your use of such tricks, you need to search your heart and mind for the cause. Nine times in 10, to find an explanation for your burnout is to find a solution for it. In my experience, the more tenacious episodes of burnout are caused by a loss of enthusiasm for the goal I'm currently chasing, or by the lack of an exciting goal. More than once, I've put an instantaneous end to a rather severe loss of motivation by coming up with a new goal. When you get the training blahs, let your imagination dream up various ideas for new challenges and see if one doesn't light your fire.

Other potential causes of lasting burnout are stress in other areas of life and overtraining. In either case, you probably need to take a little time off from serious training. This can be psychologically difficult. You fear the loss of fitness; you worry that you may never get the fire back. Such feelings are natural enough, but the reality is that you cannot continue to train hard without the will to do so. Remember, triathlon is voluntary!

Training Setbacks

Rarely does a triathlete's training cycle go totally according to plan. Even the winners of the major triathlon championships each year win despite having suffered some kind of setback—an illness, an injury, a family emergency —along the way. Understanding and accepting this reality, even expecting setbacks, will alone take you a long way toward dealing with each individual setback you encounter with minimal anguish.

Another effective tool for minimizing the stress associated with training setbacks is to fix the problems. This advice may sound stupidly obvious, but actually it is quite common for setbacks to briefly, or even not so briefly, paralyze athletes with frustration, so that not only does the situation cause more emotional torment than it needs to, but the problem itself becomes worse and lasts longer than it must. Neuropsychologists have learned that taking action—*any* responsive action—in a crisis alters brain chemistry in such a way as to lessen feelings of stress, anxiety, and depression. But not every person is equally quick to take action in a crisis. If you're inclined toward paralysis when calamity strikes, take note of this fact, and next time, do something!

Triathlon As Therapy

Life is not easy. For all its beauty and magic, life is filled with frustrations, mishaps, loss, and outright tragedy for even the most fortunate among us. Remaining happy despite life's vicissitudes requires strength. I am deeply convinced that the pursuit of endurance sports is potentially one of the most powerful sources of psychological strength that exists. It would be a shame for you or anyone to waste this potential.

Being a triathlete can benefit your overall mental well-being in the following way: As a simplified and self-contained microcosm of life, it can serve as *practice* for life, in a perfectly literal sense. As we all know, life is messy. It is fast-paced, it cannot be put on pause or set aside, and there's always a lot happening simultaneously. Sports are far tidier, yet they manifest the essential features of life (goals, rules, obstacles, plans, and hard work) and consequently the same mental skills that help one succeed in sports (motivation, determination, and so forth) also help one succeed in life. The process of preparing for and testing oneself in competition presents a terrific opportunity to develop these skills within a context that is somewhat separate from life and then apply these skills to life's challenges.

Notice I said "opportunity" and not "guarantee." The transposition of mental skills from sports to life in general is not automatic. It is possible, for example, to cultivate great confidence in the pursuit of triathlon goals and still have little confidence in the pursuit of anything else. Generalizing the mental skills you cultivate as a triathlete requires that you make a conscious effort in this direction. I strongly encourage you to make this effort. Having noticed how staying loose and playful helps your triathlon performance, try to loosen up more in your pursuit of career success. Having observed how paying attention to your body's need for rest benefits your fitness, try to be more self-observant in relation to the various mental stressors you face in life and make sure you get adequate rest from these as well. In short, view every lesson learned in triathlon as a metaphor.

On a less abstract level, individual workouts benefit one's mental health by relieving stress and tension and promoting feelings of well-being. Every exercise enthusiast knows this from experience, and in recent years the reality of this effect has been confirmed by scientific discoveries concerning its hormonal and neurological basis. But as with triathlon's potential to serve as a learning tool, workouts do not automatically relieve stress and tension and enhance feelings of well-being. It depends on the context. When completing a workout becomes yet another hassle in a hectic day, when you lack the energy needed to perform well in and enjoy a workout, or when you take a workout too seriously (for example by refusing to be satisfied by the workout unless you achieve certain split times), the potential mental health benefits of the workout can be nullified. And when spoiled workouts become a pattern, being a triathlete in itself can become bad for your mental health instead of good. Do what is needed so that you can enjoy most workouts, whether this means making more time for them, training a little less, or giving yourself the occasional attitude adjustment.

CHAPTER 10

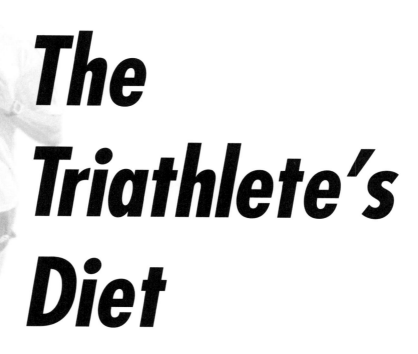

The Triathlete's Diet

One of my training partners, we'll call him Tim, is a very talented triathlete who eats four or five fast food hamburgers a week, and his other meals aren't much better. He maintains this diet simply because he likes junk food best and figures that with all the exercise he gets, it makes no difference what he swallows. I'll grant that it doesn't make a *visible* difference, but I'm convinced that Tim's already excellent performances in triathlon would be substantially better if he ate properly.

Triathlon is not an excuse to eat whatever you want. On the contrary, given the demands we place upon our bodies in daily training and our desire to perform to the best of our potential in the occasional race, we triathletes have even more reason to eat properly than nonathletes. Yes, exercise does to a degree counter the health impact of various nutritional excesses such as cholesterol consumption, but this doesn't mean excessive cholesterol does triathletes any good. It just does slightly less and/or different harm than it does nonathletes.

This is not to say that a healthy diet for a triathlete is identical to a healthy diet for a nonathlete. Due to our high activity level, we triathletes have special nutritional needs, which include greater intake of antioxidants, carbohydrate, iron, and water than less active people need. There are also the matters of nutrition before, during, and after workouts and races, representing a special area of concern for our kind.

By maintaining appropriate nutrition habits you will have better workouts, recover faster, build fitness faster, sleep better, feel better, and race more successfully than you will if you do not eat right. The objec-

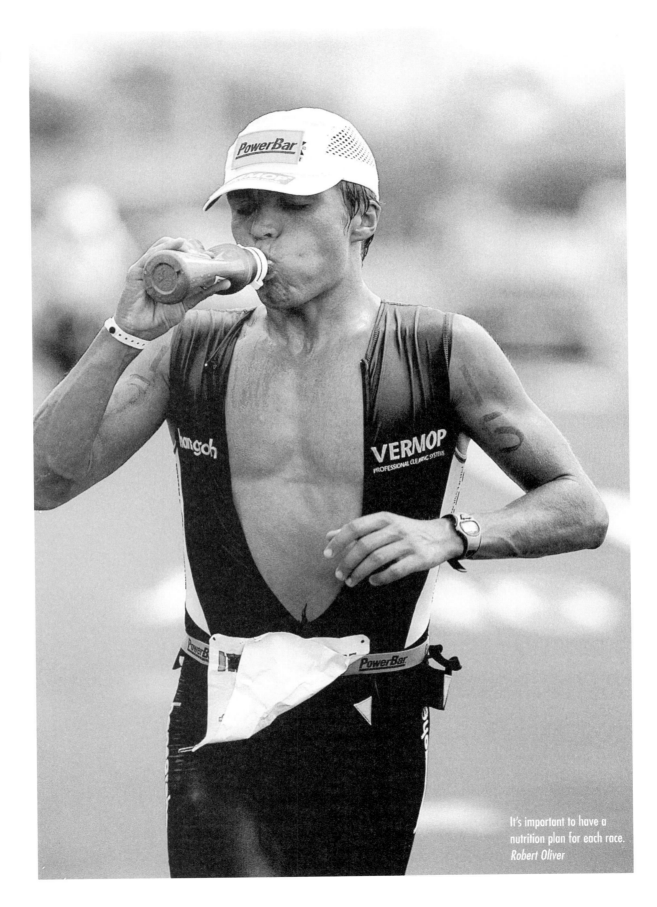

It's important to have a
nutrition plan for each race.
Robert Oliver

tive of this chapter is to tell you all you need to know in order to enjoy these worthy benefits of smart triathlon nutrition.

Everyday Nutrition

As we all know, nutrition is complex. However, if your goal is simply to know how best to fuel your triathlon lifestyle, and not necessarily to know the whole why behind the how, things are not so complex. In fact, I can reduce everything you need to know about daily nutrition for endurance performance to five basic guidelines: eat whole foods, eat a balance of foods, replace what you burn, eat for consistent energy, and stay well hydrated. Let's look at each of these guidelines.

Eat Whole Foods

Practically speaking, whole foods are foods that have not been modified from their natural state, or have been modified only a little bit, for example through cooking. Foods that *have* been significantly modified are classified as processed foods. For example, cherries are a whole food. Cherry soda is processed.

Not all forms of processing are bad. Pasteurization, for example, is a way of processing certain foods that makes them safer to eat. But most forms of processing that you cannot do with standard kitchen supplies at home make foods substantially less nutritious, and sometimes downright unhealthy. Specifically, processing foods tends to remove vital nutrients that our bodies need and introduce new substances that do not exist in nature and frequently act as toxins inside us.

Among the most commonly processed foods in the American diet are the grains we eat in baked goods and in the forms of various sugars. Grains are processed in order to speed up the manufacture of baked foods and to make them longer lasting and more appealing in taste and texture (to some palates). However, when grains are put through the process of refinement, they are stripped of their outer bran, which has all the nutrients, and they are stripped of their inner germ, which has all the fiber, so all that's left is the starchy endosperm, which is rich in carbohydrate but not much else.

The vitamin enrichment that is often done to make up for such tampering scarcely even begins to reverse the damage, largely because it cannot replace lost phytonutrients, which exist only in whole plant foods and are believed to promote health in many (mostly unknown) ways. There's a growing amount of evidence to suggest that it's not so much any one nutrient but the particular balance of many nutrients in whole foods that makes them good for us. That's not something we can re-create in the laboratory.

Processed oils are also widely used and are even less healthy. Extra-virgin olive oil is currently the only unrefined bottled oil sold on the mass market. All other bottled oils are processed in ways that remove important nutrients (including lecithin and chlorophyll) and damage a small fraction of the oil molecules, making them potentially toxic. Oils used in many packaged baked goods and snack foods and in restaurant frying are put through another process called hydrogenation. This process turns healthy, unsaturated fats into saturated and trans fats, which have been linked to heart attack, diabetes, stroke, aneurysm, weakened immune system, liver dysfunction, reproductive problems, lower IQ, prostate cancer, and breast cancer.

Dozens more food types contain unnatural ingredients as well. Many of these, such as the sodium-based preservatives used in a wide variety of products, also have known health consequences (e.g., hypertension). Others may or may not be harmful—they just haven't been studied. But it's safe to assume that any ingredient you eat that doesn't exist in nature, including colorings, flavorings, preservatives, and other additives will do you no good. At the very best, processed ingredients limit your health simply by taking the place of whole food ingredients your body knows what to do with. For example, a person who drinks soda instead of fruit juice or milk is likely to get significantly less nutrition each day than a person who avoids soda.

The nutrient density of whole foods makes them preferable for athletes, too. The demands of hard endurance training tend to deplete the body of a wide range of nutrients and create a greater need for other nutrients such as antioxidants (more on this in a moment). It is important therefore that, as a triathlete, you maximize the amount of useful nutrition you receive with each food calorie consumed, and the best way to accomplish this is by maintaining a diet rich in whole foods.

Don't think about avoiding processed foods so much as prioritizing whole foods. Denial is shaky ground for a better diet. Start by getting most of your calories each day from foods that are clearly whole in nature, such as fresh fruits and vegetables, fish, and nuts. Use only extra-virgin olive oil for cooking and limit your consumption of refined sugars and foods containing "enriched" flour, "partially hydrogenated vegetable oil," and "vegetable shortening." When you're in doubt about a food's relative wholeness, compare the list of ingredients to a recipe for the same food. They should match.

And if you really want to get serious about whole foods, start paying attention to the food *your food eats*. When a chicken lives in the wild, it eats live foods that it chooses. When it lives in a chicken factory, it is fed processed feed that has been made with shelf life in mind. Since the chicken is made out of food, and the eggs that it lays are made out of food, the quality of the food that it has been fed is reflected in its meat and in its eggs. The same pattern holds for pigs, cattle, and even things like farmed salmon. Since it's hard to come by meat from animals raised on all-natural foods, I recommend using ocean seafood as a primary protein source.

The one important exception to the whole foods rule for triathletes is the case of exercise nutrition. During exercise, man-made ergogenic (energy-producing) supplements are preferable to any kind of real food. I'm talking about sports drinks, gels, and to a lesser extent, energy bars. These supplements—the good ones, anyway—have been designed to provide exactly what your body needs during strenuous physical activity (mainly water, electrolytes, and carbohydrate) and nothing more that could hinder the delivery of these things to your muscles. I'll have more to say about nutrition during exercise in a later section of this chapter.

What about other supplements? Taking a daily multivitamin as insurance, not as a real-food substitute, is a sensible practice, especially if you have known vitamin or mineral deficiencies. As for the various sports supplements that are widely used, none has proven itself to the degree that its use should be encouraged. Many runners and triathletes take glucosamine and chondroitin sulfate supplements to strengthen the cartilage, but the best evidence indicates that these runners and triathletes are wasting their money. Some triathletes take creatine monohydrate to gain muscle strength, but such strength gains, even when they do occur, do not translate into improved endurance performance. In short, while I won't rule out the possibility of some must-have supplement for endurance athletes arising in the future, it is clear that none is known today.

Eat a Balance of Foods

No single food provides every nutrient we need. In fact, no single food even comes close. For this reason, it is important that we consistently eat a variety of foods in our diet. Making good use of this advice requires that you have a general understanding of the basic food categories. It makes the most sense to categorize foods by the types of nutrients they provide. Ordered from what we need in the greatest amount to what we need in the least amount, these categories are: grains; fruits and vegetables; nuts, seeds, and plant oils; and animal foods. Here's what each category provides:

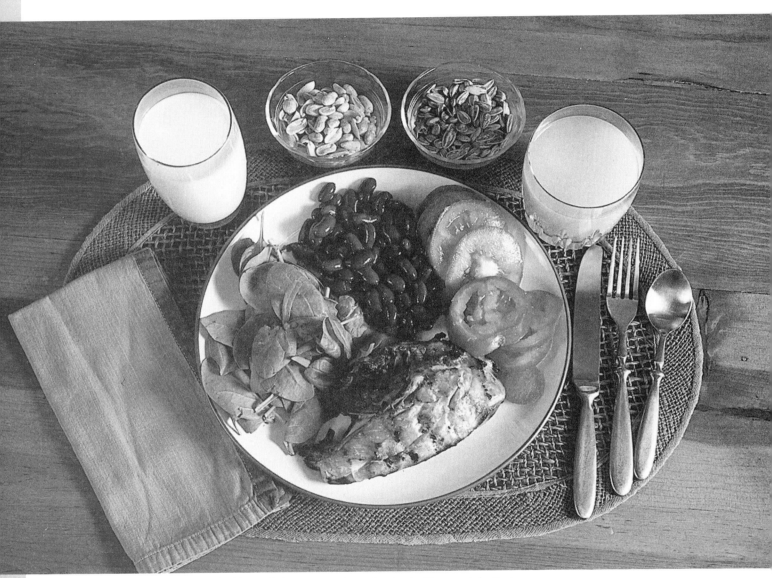

With a little effort, you can have healthy meals that taste even better than less healthy ones. *Luke Harrig*

Grains

The most important type of nutrient provided in grains such as brown rice, whole wheat, and whole oats is the macronutrient carbohydrate. Grains—and they should virtually always be whole grains—are rich in carbohydrate, which should account for about 60 percent of the calories in a triathlete's diet. For this reason, I recommend that you eat a whole grain food at virtually every meal, including snacks. Whole grains are also high in fiber, which helps the processing and elimination of waste; vitamins such as B_1 (thiamine) and B_2 (riboflavin), which assist carbohydrate, fat, and protein metabolism; and minerals such as magnesium, which assist enzyme activation, nerve and muscle function, and calcium and potassium balance.

Fruits and Vegetables

As a general category, fruits and vegetables provide every kind of vitamin and mineral our bodies need, as well as countless useful phytonutrients, some known, most still unknown. But of course not all fruits and vegetables are the same. Each provides a lot of some nutrients and not a lot of others. And so your balanced diet must also contain a balance of different fruits and vegetables. Scarfing five bananas a day won't cut it.

Make sure to include citrus fruits, known for their vitamin C content; green leafy vegetables, which offer, among other things, the iron that is essential to forming the oxygen transporters hemoglobin in the blood and myoglobin in the muscles; and legumes, such as various types of beans, which are loaded with fiber and folate, used in protein metabolism, cell division, and red blood cell formation. You should eat fruits and vegetables five times a day, at least, which may sound onerous, but keep in mind that such things as a glass of 100 percent fruit juice and a handful of dried fruit count as full servings. A nice big salad can easily account for two servings.

Nuts, Seeds, and Plant Oils

This food category is basically shorthand for sources of healthy vegetable fats. Our bodies need fat for the formation of cell membranes and hormones, for brain and nervous system function, and for energy. Good sources of healthy vegetable fats include all kinds of seeds and nuts, the oils derived from them, olives and olive oil, soybeans, avocados, and corn. Be sure to eat a few healthy fat foods every day.

Animal Foods

Human beings don't need animal foods at all, and as you know, in our society many people do choose to eschew them for reasons ranging from health to politics. Certain animal foods should be avoided or mostly avoided by everyone. However, many animal foods are quite healthful for most people, and it's a little easier to maintain a balanced diet by eating certain animal foods than it is as a vegetarian.

Meats, fish, eggs, and dairy foods are all excellent sources of protein, the main structural ingredient of all cells and enzymes. Protein should account for about 15 percent of the calories in a triathlete's diet. In addition, various particular types of animal foods are good sources of a variety of other nutrients. For example, beef is high in the minerals iron and zinc, dairy foods are high in the mineral calcium, and certain kinds of fish are high in essential fatty acids.

If your cholesterol ratio is less than ideal, you may wish to avoid animal foods containing a lot of saturated fat (including whole milk dairy foods and many cuts of beef, pork, and lamb), which increases "bad" cholesterol production. And we should all try to avoid animal foods loaded with hormones, antibiotics, and God knows what else they use in animal food factories these days (e.g., supermarket chicken and eggs). The best animal foods are deep-sea fish, organic dairy foods, and free-range and wild game meats. Two such foods a day are plenty for omnivores who get enough whole grains, legumes, and nuts, seeds, and oils.

Replace What You Burn

It is normal for beginning triathletes to lose weight as a result of burning calories during workouts and increasing their resting metabolism. In a few cases, very skinny beginning triathletes may initially gain weight in the form of lean muscle tissue. In all other cases, triathletes should consume the same number of calories they burn and maintain a fairly consistent body weight.

There are two ways to make sure you are in fact maintaining this balance. The simplest is to monitor your weight by stepping onto the scale once a week or so. If you find you're gaining more than a little weight, or gaining it gradually but steadily, you're consuming too many calories; if you're losing weight, you're consuming too few calories. The second option is to count the number of calories you consume on a daily basis and estimate the number of calories you burn. Web sites such as Active.com provide tools that allow you to do this fairly easily. I wouldn't bother with this more involved measure, though, unless you find that you are gaining or losing weight and you want to figure out why. In this case, you'll need to figure out not just your total daily caloric consumption but also your consumption by macronutrient, as these numbers will give you information about which foods you need more or less of. As a triathlete, you should maintain a diet comprised of approximately 60 percent carbohydrate, 25 percent fat, and 15 percent protein.

Naturally, the primary determinant of how many calories you need at any given time is your training volume. The more you train, the more calories you burn and need to replace. Therefore, expect your caloric and carbohydrate needs to fluctuate over the course of a training cycle, and act accordingly. Generally, when you are increasing your training load, you can rely on your appetite to motivate additional consumption, but sometimes when you decrease your training load (as during tapering or the off-season), your appetite might not immediately follow suit, in which case you'll need to consciously reduce intake.

Eat for Consistent Energy

It is better to have a relatively steady supply of energy throughout the day than to experience energy peaks and valleys. The peaks aren't so bad, actually, but the valleys are, and the latter tend to follow the former. Crashing is disruptive enough for nonathletes, but for triathletes it's an outright nuisance because we need to count on having adequate energy for solid workouts once and often twice a day.

The two practices you can rely on to give you consistent energy throughout the day are eating frequently and getting the majority of your carbohydrate calories from what are called low-glycemic carbohydrates. The energy crashes we tend to experience in certain parts of the day (late morning and mid-afternoon are the most common times) are usually caused by low blood glucose levels. The longer it's been since you last consumed carbohydrate, the lower your blood glucose level is likely to be. Clearly, then, eating frequently (and in particular, eating carbohydrate frequently) is a way to prevent crash-level drops in blood glucose from occurring. Endurance sports nutrition experts generally recommend eating five to six times a day: breakfast, mid-morning snack, lunch, mid-afternoon snack, dinner, and for those who need it, an evening snack. Each of these meals should include carbohydrate.

Some carbohydrates provide more lasting energy than others. Those that provide more lasting energy are known as low-glycemic carbohydrates. These carbohydrates are digested more slowly than their high-glycemic counterparts. However, bear in mind that some foods that contain low-glycemic carbohydrates have so little *total* carbohydrate in them that they're no better as a lasting energy source than many foods containing only simple sugars. Peanuts are a good example of such a food—they're quite good for you, but not as an energy source. Examples of foods that are low-glycemic *and* rich in total carbohydrate are whole grain foods, some fruits including pears and apples, many kinds of beans, and a variety of breakfast cereals.

There's also a way to effectively turn high-glycemic carbohydrate foods into low-glycemic foods: namely, by eating them with protein or fat, or both. The presence of protein and fat tends to slow the delivery of carbohydrate into the bloodstream. For example, white rice is a relatively fast-burning carbohydrate-rich food, but when combined with beans and/or fish or meat, it provides more lasting energy.

Stay Well Hydrated

I won't teach you anything new by telling you that adequate water intake is critical for good health. We all know that water is an essential nutrient for maintaining blood volume, lubricating cells, ridding the body of metabolic wastes, and so forth. And yet, according to a source as knowledgeable as longtime Hawaii Ironman medical director Bob Laird, M.D., a great many triathletes are chronically dehydrated. This is because triathletes really have to drink *a lot* of water every day to make up for all the water they lose through perspiration in their workouts. Merely making an effort to stay fully hydrated won't suffice. It must be an ingrained habit.

So, just how much water do you need? This depends on factors that include your weight, the weather, other dietary considerations such as caffeine intake (which increases water needs), and, of course, your training volume. The *average* person requires roughly one ounce of water per kilogram (2.2 pounds) of body weight on a daily basis. Athletes generally need a little more. Another guideline is to simply drink as much water as you can tolerate without feeling bloated and sloshy. I sip from a water bottle literally all day long and I've never felt any indication that I may be drinking too much.

Individual Needs

Every person requires the same basic set of nutrients for life, health, and fitness. However, individual persons need different amounts of these nutrients. Each human being is metabolically unique, and consequently each of us must fine-tune our diets within the universal parameters of human needs in order to find our personal, optimal diet—which itself will need to evolve as we ourselves change. Obvious examples of the need to fine-tune are cases of food allergies and intolerances such as those that many people in our society have to lactose and wheat gluten.

But most examples are subtler, like the many gradations in vitamin and mineral requirements that different individuals have.

Triathletes have a second set of individual nutritional needs beyond everyday nutrition—namely, workout and race nutrition. For example, individual triathletes lose electrolytes at different rates during exercise, and those who lose more sometimes have to supplement their sports drink intake with salt tablets during long, hot races. Some triathletes experience bowel troubles during racing unless they are very careful about what they eat beforehand. Some triathletes are able to ingest more carbohydrate during exercise than others. And so forth.

How do you determine your individual needs? For everyday nutrition, there are two methods that work well. The first is to have doctors test you for food allergies and intolerances and for vitamin and mineral deficiencies. Since particular deficiencies (e.g., iron) are common among endurance athletes, this is something your doctor should readily do for you. A less precise but far more comprehensive way to determine your individual nutritional needs is through evaluative dietary record keeping. The general idea here is to record when, what, and how much you eat and drink and how these things affect your subsequent functioning and workouts. If you keep this habit up long enough, you can isolate patterns, for better or worse, test them, and then make permanent any changes that seem to help. Table 10.1 suggests a format for evaluative dietary record keeping.

Of course, in order for the dietary record strategy to pay dividends, you need to fiddle with your eating patterns. Even if you feel good most of the time and have confidence in your diet already, there is fiddling you can do. The first modifications you should try are those that would seem to correct obvious problems in your diet. For example, if you're not eating breakfast, you can try eating breakfast. If you eat a lot of refined sugar, you can try reducing your refined sugar intake. Once you've taken care of the gross deviations from nutritional good sense, you can begin to test hunches and recommendations you take from trusted nutrition authorities. For example, perhaps you've long suspected that your body has trouble processing dairy foods, yet you've continued to eat them because you like them and you've been able to live with the symptoms (so far). In this case, see how you feel without dairy in your diet for a couple of weeks (but of course make sure to take in compensating sources of vitamin D and calcium).

In order to determine your during-exercise nutritional needs, start by following the general recommendations provided in the next section. Evaluate how these refueling patterns work for you by taking note of var-

Sample Evaluative Dietary Record Format

	Two Hours Later	Subsequent Workout
Meal 1: (When? What? How much?)	Appetite? Energy? Mental Clarity? Mood?	Energy? Gastrointestinal troubles? Focus? Attitude?
Meal 2		
Meal 3		
Meal 4		
Meal 5		
Meal 6	Sleep?	
Table 10.1		

ious effects. Problems to watch out for are bonking (running out of energy late in a workout or race), overheating, nausea, bloating, cramping, and bowel situations. A tendency to bonk (if not due to unwise pacing) indicates a need to consume more carbohydrate; a tendency to overheat indicates a need for more water and/or electrolyte intake; nausea and bloating are generally caused by consuming too many calories or too much fluid at once, or by eating too soon or too much before exercise; and cramping can also be caused by eating too much or too soon before exercise and by depletion of the electrolyte potassium.

Some nutritional needs are neither universal nor individual but are, rather, particular to endurance athletes as a group. The high level of carbohydrate intake mentioned above is the most celebrated one. Fewer triathletes are aware that endurance athletes also need more protein than nonathletes due to the muscle protein breakdown that occurs daily in workouts. Sedentary adults require about 0.5 gram per pound of body weight of protein daily, whereas triathletes require between 0.7 and 1.0 gram per pound of body weight, depending on training volume. Beyond these macronutrients, deficiencies in the minerals iron and zinc are common among endurance athletes, and especially female endurance athletes. A deficiency in iron particularly can have a devastating effect on fitness. As a triathlete, you should eat plenty of iron- and zinc-rich foods such as beans and whole grains, and take a daily multivitamin with iron and zinc as insurance.

Endurance athletes also need more antioxidant vitamins and minerals than the average person. While nearly every physical adaptation associated with intensive endurance training is healthy, one notable exception is the oxidative stress incurred by athletes' tissues through exercise. Oxygen is a potent free radical. The heavy oxygen demand associated with endurance exercise causes accelerated damage to healthy cells in the body. Over time, it is believed, such damage can lead to certain degenerative diseases and speed the aging process. Vitamins A, C, and E and the mineral selenium are known to reduce oxidative stress. Again, in addition to consuming foods rich in these nutrients, you should take a daily multivitamin that contains them.

Nutrition Before Exercise

Pre-exercise nutrition is a matter of balance. On the one hand, you want to take in sufficient energy close enough to your workout or race to properly fuel the ensuing performance. On the other hand, you want to avoid the cramping, nausea, and reduced blood flow to working muscles that tend to result when you take in too much food too close to your workout or race.

The first rule for achieving this balance is to keep your body well fueled for exercise generally by consuming lots of carbohydrate and plenty of water on a daily basis. There are world-class endurance athletes who get a nervous stomach and cannot eat a breakfast before competing, but who excel anyway because they keep their bodies fully stocked with carbohydrate fuel and water through the habits they maintain before race day. You can further reduce the need to cram in calories on race morning by practicing carbohydrate loading in the three or four days preceding a triathlon. Let me say a few words about this practice before I return to the topic of guidelines for eating in the hours before workouts and races.

Endurance athletes have been practicing pre-race carbohydrate loading for more than 25 years. Even so, it is often done incorrectly. Some of us eat a heaping bowl of pasta the night before a race and call this carbo loading. (It's not.) Others continue to practice 1970s-style carbo loading, in which the actual loading phase is preceded by an unpleasant, potentially hazardous, and not altogether necessary carbohydrate depletion phase. And still others are simply vague on the details: how long the loading period should last, how much carbohydrate they should eat, and so forth. Here's the straight dope on carbo loading.

The rationale behind the practice of pre-race carbohydrate loading is simple. In long endurance events, glucose (a product of carbohydrate breakdown) is the primary fuel used for the repetitive muscle contractions that propel the body forward. This fuel is obtained from the blood and from a substance very similar to glucose called glycogen that is stored in skeletal muscle and in the liver. The more blood glucose and muscle and liver glycogen your body can make available for energy during races, the longer you will be able to delay fatigue. The way to maximize blood glucose is to take in carbohydrates before the race, in the form of a sensible pre-race meal, and during exercise, in the form of sports drinks, gels, and possibly energy bars or other snacks.

There are three ways to maximize muscle and liver glycogen storage. The first is to train. Improvement in the muscles' capacity to store muscle glycogen is one of the primary effects of endurance training. The second way is to taper. Individual workouts deplete glycogen supplies. By greatly reducing your training volume in the days before a race, your glycogen supplies will naturally top off. A third way is to increase carbohydrate consumption in the few days before a long race. Many studies have shown that three days of supranormal carbohydrate intake effectively increase both muscle glycogen storage and performance in events lasting 90 minutes or more.

Many different carbo loading protocols have been tried and tested. The primary variables involved are the length of the loading period, the baseline level of carbohydrate consumption preceding it, the amount by which carbohydrate consumption increases during loading, total calories consumed, and whether the loading period is preceded by a period of carbohydrate depletion. This last factor has been the source of the greatest controversy. The original glycogen depletion protocol called for athletes to drastically reduce carbohydrate consumption (down to 10 percent of total calories) for the first three days of race week and perform intensive workouts on these days to further diminish stored glycogen. The next three days called for massive carbohydrate intake (as much as 90 percent of total calories) and very light workouts.

The rationale for the depletion phase is that the body naturally tends to sponge up vital nutrients that it is deprived of for a period of time. Studies have shown that this protocol does in fact lead to substantially increased glycogen storage. However, carbohydrate is indeed a vital nutrient, and depleting it can lead to severe fatigue, irritability, and even sickness and injury. If you've ever done it, you know it's not fun—especially when you try to work out intensively with so little fuel in the tank.

Fortunately, other studies have shown that you can increase glycogen storage significantly without first depleting it. A newer carbo loading protocol based on this research calls for athletes to eat a normal diet (that is, normal for an endurance athlete) containing 60 percent carbohydrate until three days before racing, and then switch over to a 70 percent carbohydrate diet for these final three days, plus race morning. In terms of exercise, the protocol suggests one last longer workout a week from race day followed by increasingly shorter workouts throughout race week. It's simple, it's nonexcruciating, and it works. Admittedly, some scientists and athletes still swear that the depletion protocol is more effective, but if it is, the difference is slight and probably not worth the suffering and inherent risks.

Note that you should increase your carbohydrate intake not by increasing your total caloric intake, but rather by reducing fat and protein intake in an amount that equals or slightly exceeds the amount of carbohydrate you add. Combining less training with more calories could result in last-minute weight gain that will only slow you down. Be aware, too, that for every gram of carbohydrate the body stores, it also stores three to five grams of water, which leads many athletes to feel bloated by the end of a three-day loading period. The extra stored water is not a bad thing, though, considering that dehydration is as big an issue as glycogen depletion in long races.

As for figuring out how much carbohydrate you're eating, it's easiest to count grams. In your normal diet, eating six to seven grams of carbohydrate per kilogram (2.2 pounds) of body weight will put you in the right percentage range. During the loading period, you should consume 10 to 11 grams of carbohydrate per kilogram of body weight. You can determine how many grams of carbohydrate various foods contain by reading labels and by consulting resources such as *The Complete Book of Food Counts*. As always, use high-quality carbohydrate sources such as whole grains rather than poor ones like cookies.

One may ask why endurance athletes should not eat this loading volume of carbohydrate all the time. The reason is that it crowds out the other macronutrients, protein and fat, which your body also needs. Just three days of relatively reduced protein and fat intake will do you no harm, but more certainly would.

Even if you do practice carbo loading, it's best if you can eat some kind of meal within one to four hours of racing. The same guideline holds for workouts, for which you will never carbo load. If your last meal before exercise falls close to four hours out, it can be, and indeed should, be larger—up to 1,000 calories. If it falls one hour out, it has to be fairly small—300 to 400 calories. In either case, the meal should be high in carbohydrate, moderate to low in protein, low in fat and fiber, and devoid of gas-producing foods such as onions and beans. Within these parameters, find the protocol that works best for you by experimenting. Generally, triathletes can get away with eating more food closer to cycling workouts than running workouts, while swim workouts tend to fall in between.

Your pre-workout meals can be a little less perfect than your pre-race meals, which should be as perfect as you can make them. Because most triathlons take place early in the morning, eating more than two hours beforehand can be impractical. Sleep is no less important than fuel. So, developing your ideal pre-race meal is a matter of figuring out what you can best tolerate two hours before racing. Once you've found this meal, stick with it.

Nutrition During Exercise

The purpose of taking in nutrients during workouts and races is essentially to refuel muscles. The benefits of replenishing energy and fluid during exercise (be it training or racing) include better performance, delay of fatigue, and even reduction in muscle damage. There are two components of muscle fueling: fluid and energy. Let's first talk about the fluid component.

As you've been told a thousand times, the human body is made of mostly water, and indeed triathletes are even more watery than nonathletes due to our greater blood volume and lean tissue composition (fat is the least watery tissue in the body). Water is involved in virtually every bodily process, from lubricating tissue cells to flushing wastes from the body. At rest, you lose a little water through breathing and sweating and substantially more through urination. During exercise, however, the rate of water loss through sweating increases dramatically, as perspiration is the body's main cooling mechanism in adults. Working muscles generate heat, which your blood whisks away and carries to capillaries near the surface of the skin, where the heat-carrying water content of the blood is released onto the surface of the body. Cooled blood then continues to circulate.

It works pretty well, but this cooling system has limitations. First, the longer it continues, the less effective it becomes, as the water content of the blood continually decreases. The dehydration process renders the blood not only less able to conduct heat, but also less able to do everything else it's supposed to do, like carry nutrients to tissue cells. In addition, water is not the only vital nutrient lost in sweat; also lost are the minerals sodium, chloride, potassium, and magnesium, collectively known as electrolytes because they conduct the body's electrical signals. As the electrolytes become depleted, the body becomes less efficient in transmitting nerve and motor impulses and maintaining proper fluid balance.

As little as a 2 percent loss of body fluids, which can occur in as little as an hour of moderately intense exercise, can have a detrimental impact on endurance performance. Hence, triathletes should try to fully replace the water and electrolyte losses that occur during exercise. However, it is seldom possible to achieve this ideal of complete compensation, as the human body is simply not designed for rapid rehydration. When too much fluid is consumed, bloating and nausea can result. As a general rule, then, you should consume as much fluid as you can tolerate during workouts and competitions. Fluid tolerance while bicycling is always higher (more than double) than fluid tolerance while running. Triathletes can often increase their tolerance for fluid consumption during exercise simply by practicing it consistently.

Different people lose fluids at different rates during exercise. You can estimate your own standard rate of sweat loss by weighing yourself (preferably on a scale with pounds and ounces) immediately before and after a typical workout and figuring in fluid consumed and urine excreted during the workout. For example, suppose a given athlete loses 15 ounces in a 60-minute workout during which he neither drinks nor urinates. This athlete should try to replace 15 ounces of fluid for each hour of exercise (but can expect to be able to replace only 80 percent of this amount—about 12 ounces). Quantifying fluid loss in this way can be quite eye-opening for endurance athletes, but I need to emphasize that regardless of the number you come up with, your procedure should be the same: to take in as much fluid as you can tolerate in all workouts lasting an hour or more. This is especially true in higher environmental temperatures and higher exercise intensities, which increase the rate of fluid loss. Note that the fuller the stomach is, the faster it empties, so it's a good idea to drink immediately before workouts and to drink small amounts frequently during exercise to keep stomach volume as high as possible.

Always use a sports drink for rehydration during exercise. Water is not sufficient, because drinking water does not replace electrolyte losses that occur through perspiration (nor does it address carbohydrate depletion, which I'll address momentarily). Some athletes prefer water because they feel it quenches their thirst better, but the fact that sports drinks are less effective in quenching the thirst sensation represents another one of their advantages—their sodium content actually stimulates thirst and motivates you to drink more. Rates of electrolyte loss also vary from one athlete to the next, but in general it is easier to fully compensate for electrolyte losses during exercise than for water losses. Most sports drinks are formulated to provide electrolytes and water in the proper ratio to make up for the effects of perspiration. Failure to take in sufficient amounts of electrolytes during prolonged exercise can result in a condition called hyponatremia characterized by dangerouly low sodium levels in the blood.

As I've mentioned, the primary fuel sources for moderate- to high-intensity exercise are glycogen stored in the muscles and liver and glucose carried to working muscles through the blood. Both glycogen and glucose are products of carbohydrate breakdown, and for this reason they are often referred to collectively as "carbohydrate fuel." Blood glucose is available in more limited amounts than muscle and liver glycogen, but it can be replenished much more rapidly. It takes many hours to replenish glycogen through carbohydrate consumption, while it takes only about 20 minutes for the sugars consumed in a sports drink to pass through the stomach and become broken down into glucose in the bloodstream. This is why consuming carbohydrate during exercise is essential for prolonging endurance. While you cannot consume enough carbohydrate to completely halt the use of glycogen for energy, you can consume enough to slow its depletion significantly.

Studies have consistently shown that consuming the proper carbohydrate sources (namely simple sugars and polymers such as glucose and maltodextrin) in the proper amounts can delay fatigue in endurance athletes. The greatest performance benefits result when 60 to 80 grams of carbohydrate are consumed per hour of intense exercise. In most athletes, the gastrointestinal tract cannot absorb carbohydrate at a rate exceeding 1.2 grams per minute, and when greater amounts are consumed, gastrointestinal distress often occurs. Consuming fewer than 60 grams of carbohydrate per hour fails to take advantage of the glycogen-sparing effect that results when blood glucose levels are maximized during exercise. Sports drinks that are formulated to take care of athletes' fluid, electrolyte, and carbohydrate needs should contain 6 to 8 percent carbohydrate to ensure that carbohydrate is delivered at the appropriate rate.

Sports drinks are ideal and sufficient for your nutritional needs in most training and racing situations. Carry an adequate supply with you, or have an adequate supply available, for all workouts lasting longer than 45 minutes. You can achieve similar results by combining energy gels such as ClifShot and GU with water (but be aware that some energy gels do not contain electrolytes); however, most athletes find the sports drinks more convenient. Combining energy gel use with sports drink consumption is generally not a good idea, as the heavy carbohydrate load will slow down gastric emptying and delivery of nutrients to the muscles.

A few sports drinks and gels contain antioxidants such as vitamins C and E. These nutrients do not enhance performance, but they do limit the amount of free radical damage that muscle cells normally incur during workouts, and for this reason I highly recommend that you choose sports drinks and gels that contain them. Some of the newer sports drinks, such as Accelerade, also contain protein. Recent studies have shown that when a small amount protein is included in a sports drink, insulin levels remain higher during exercise and as a result, carbohydrate is delivered to the muscles more rapidly. In addition, the added protein may decrease muscle protein breakdown during exercise and accelerate post-exercise protein rebuilding. The ideal amount of protein in a sports drink is about 6 or 7 grams per 12 ounces.

In long cycling workouts and in the cycling leg of triathlons lasting longer than three hours, you may want to supplement your sports drink with the use of energy bars or possibly even "real" food. This is because you might actually get hungry during long rides and races and will want to fill some space in your rumbling gut, or because you might wish to avoid or minimize the stomach sloshing that can happen when you consume only liquids for hours on end. Whatever you choose to eat should contain mostly carbohydrate and not too much protein, fat, or fiber. I don't recommend trying to eat solid food while running unless you've got a cast iron stomach.

Also, before very long workouts and races, you may wish to take in some caffeine. There is a growing body of evidence to suggest that it can help delay fatigue of the central nervous system, which generally parallels muscle fatigue. For that matter, there is also research suggesting that caffeine can increase fat metabolism during exercise, which is a highly desirable effect and could justify the consumption of modest amounts—about two milligrams per pound of body weight—of caffeine before races of any length. However, I need to stress that we still lack *definitive* proof that caffeine can enhance endurance performance. Further, some individuals do not react well to caffeine intake. So the most I can recommend is that you try the use of caffeine before one or two lower-priority races. Take an appropriate dose of caffeine about one hour before racing in the form of a pill such as No-Doz rather than in a beverage such as coffee or soda. For whatever reason, the performance-enhancing effects of caffeine appear to be neutralized when the stimulant is not taken in a more or less pure form. Some energy gels do contain caffeine in an effective form, but usually not in sufficient amounts.

You should go into each race with a precise nutrition plan. You need to know what you're going to drink, and possibly eat, and when, and how. Know where aid stations are located and what they offer. Know how you're going to carry the nutrition you will carry on the bike and possibly on the run. Of course, your plan should be inherently flexible, so that it is able to meet your needs regardless of how you feel during various stages of the race, which is impossible to predict. But there's a difference between having a flexible plan and winging it.

The best ways to come up with the right nutrition plan for any given race are through experience in training and racing and through observing what works for others. No triathlete nails his or her nutrition the first time. In the beginning, you need to simply follow general recommendations. In the course of following these guidelines, try to identify problems and limitations associated with your nutrition strategy and then test likely solutions in subsequent training and racing. Observing others' methods will give you an infinite supply of new things to try, from different sports drink options to clever ways of affixing gel packets to your bike. Just don't try the silly ideas.

Nutrition for Recovery

The area of post-exercise nutrition was largely ignored until just a few years ago, when new knowledge about the physiology of recovery made it an area of intense interest almost overnight. In a nutshell, what we've learned is that consuming the right nutrients in the right amounts shortly after completing exercise can greatly enhance and accelerate your recovery, which in turn will help you perform better in your next workout.

There are three things you need to recover from after a workout or race: glycogen depletion in the muscles and liver, fluid loss, and muscle tissue damage. Restocking glycogen stores is a slow process. With normal nutrition intake, it can take your body as many as 48 hours to top off muscle and liver glycogen after a race or particularly hard workout. But you can kick-start this process by taking in at least 60 grams of carbohydrate within an hour of completing exercise. During this period, your body is able to replenish glycogen at almost twice the normal rate, so it's important to take advantage of this window of opportunity.

As I mentioned above, it is generally impossible to replace fluids at the same rate at which they're lost through perspiration during exercise. Thus you are unavoidably left in a state of fluid deficit after each work-out. You need to eliminate this deficit as quickly as possible by drinking water and/or a sports drink. If you drink water, make sure to eat something that contains sodium and potassium, such as an energy bar, to replace the electrolytes you've also lost in your sweat. A sports drink—and especially one formulated especially for recovery—can take care of your initial post-exercise carbohydrate needs in addition to your water and electrolyte needs.

In order to kick-start the muscle repair process, you should also take in a small amount of protein in the first hour after working out or racing. Taking in too much protein will slow the glycogen replenishment process, however. One gram of protein for every four grams of carbohydrate you consume is about right. There are some sports recovery drinks that contain protein, too. Since appetite is commonly suppressed following exercise, these drinks offer a practical way to get all the nutrition you need after training or racing, but they're not essential. You can get the same results with your own food and drink selections. One thing to avoid, if you do choose to chow down soon after cooling down, is fat, which will also slow the absorption of the carbohydrate you need most at this time.

Eating for Endurance

Following is an example of a good day's nutritional intake for a triathlete. It is presented neither as a perfect meal plan nor as ideal for every triathlete. In fact, it's more or less just what I ate yesterday. Nevertheless, this menu provides a basic template that can serve as a starting point for any endurance athlete and it shows one way, among thousands, in which the nutritional guidelines provided in this chapter can be put into delicious, satisfying practice.

BREAKFAST 7:00 A.M.

Large bowl of oatmeal with raisins, walnuts, and real maple syrup
Large glass of orange juice
Multivitamin
Coffee (black)

MID-MORNING SNACK

Apple
Several handfuls of salted cashews

NOON WORKOUT

12 ounces of sports drink

LUNCH

Tuna salad (made with mustard, olive oil, diced onions, and
    black pepper) on whole wheat bread with lettuce and tomato
One (6-oz.) tub of low-fat organic peach yogurt
A handful of olive oil potato chips
12-oz. bottle of apple juice

MID-AFTERNOON SNACK

Energy bar
8 carrot sticks

FIVE O'CLOCK WORKOUT

12 ounces of sports drink

DINNER

Ahi tuna steak with lemon butter dill sauce
Brown rice
Steamed asparagus drizzled with olive oil
Large glass of 2 percent milk
Banana nut muffin for dessert

EVENING SNACK

Bowl of Total cereal with 2 percent milk
Banana

Triathletes and Smoothies

Y ou aren't a real triathlete unless you juice.

That's not true. What I meant to say was that juicing—by which I mean blending one's own fruit smoothies at home—is something that a great many triathletes enjoy doing, especially in triathlon's birthplace of southern California. In fact, juicing is so popular among triathletes that *Triathlete* even carried a "Smoothie of the Month" department for a while. The two activities are perfect complements to each other. Triathlon is a healthy mix of different sports, while homemade smoothies are a healthy mix of fresh fruit juices and other ingredients that serve as the perfect fuel for triathlon training.

What does it take to participate in this daily rite of the triathlon lifestyle? Not much: a blender, possibly a juicer, a few ingredients, and at least one recipe. The juicer you need only if you plan to juice vegetables and harder fruits such as apples. If you wish to use only softer fruits like berries and peaches, a blender will do the job. Or you can always buy carrot or apple juice and pour it in the blender.

A traditional smoothie has two components: a base and fruit. The base component provides volume, a different taste to mix with those of the fruits included, and possibly some nutrition that complements that which the fruit provides. Popular base ingredients are ice, milk, yogurt, ice cream, frozen yogurt, and fruit sorbet. Which one or ones you choose depends on the flavor, texture, and nutrition you desire. Bananas are a fruit that is used as a kind of base because they are cheap and have a light flavor.

The fruits that are most often used in homemade smoothies include blueberries, strawberries, cranberries, cherries, bananas, kiwifruit, cantaloupe, oranges, tangerines, and pineapples, but there are several other possibilities. You can use fresh fruit, frozen fruit, or a combination of the two. Fresh fruit is preferable when it's in season, but be aware that "fresh" fruits that appear in the supermarket out of season are less nutritious due to their having been stored for long periods of time under conditions that prevent them from ripening. Try to choose organic fruit over nonorganic. For health and environmental reasons, it's worth the extra cost.

Put your desired base and fruit choices in a blender, blend them, and you've got a smoothie. It may take a few tries before you find the blend of ingredients that tastes best and provides the best consistency—very thick, but decidedly liquid—but I can guarantee that even your failures will be pretty tasty and very good for you. If you like, you can add to your smoothie recipes any of a number of nutritional additions that home juicers like to use, from powdered enzymes to soy protein powder.

Here's my favorite homemade smoothie recipe:

The Triathlete Special

One cup 2 percent milk

One cup ice

One banana

One half-cup blueberries

One half-cup strawberries

Glossary

Absorption A process by which systems of the body recover from individual workouts and adapt to a series of workouts.

Acceleration A running drill wherein a runner begins at a moderate pace and accelerates to a sub-sprint over a distance of about 100 meters.

Active recovery Low-intensity swimming, cycling, or running for the purpose of recovering between intervals within a workout or recovering from a recent race or hard workout.

Adaptation A process whereby fitness improves as various systems of the body respond to the repeated application of stress in workouts over time.

Aero An abbreviation of "aerodynamic." An aero frame is a bike frame designed with blade-shaped tubes to minimize wind drag. Aero wheels are similarly designed bicycle wheels.

Aerobar A type of bicycle handlebar on which the rider rests his or her forearms and which is often used in triathlons.

Aerobic Refers to a process by which the body produces energy for movement by breaking down carbohydrate and fat in the presence of oxygen.

Age group A competitive division in a triathlon defined by gender and age (e.g., "female 25–29").

Age-grouper An amateur triathlete.

Agonist A muscle that contracts in order to flex or extend a joint.

Anabolic Refers to nutrients or dietary patterns that have a muscle-building effect in the body.

Anaerobic Refers to a process by which the body produces energy for movement by breaking down carbohydrate without oxygen.

Anaerobic threshold A level of exercise intensity beyond which the body cannot consume oxygen fast enough to support the energy demand. As a result, lactic acid begins to rapidly accumulate in the blood, hastening exhaustion. Also known as **lactate threshold.**

Antagonist A muscle that relaxes and stretches while one or more muscles on the opposite side of the same joint contract.

Anterior Refers to the front side of the body.

Antioxidants Nutrients that attach themselves to free radical molecules, thereby neutralizing them and preventing them from damaging tissues.

Attack To suddenly increase riding intensity on the bike in order to escape competitors, meet the challenge of a hill, or for other similar reasons.

Base phase The first of three phases in the training cycle, during which a triathlete focuses on gradually building general endurance by performing an increasing volume of low- to moderate-intensity training.

Body marking Having one's race number and age written on one's body in Magic Marker by a race official prior to the start of a triathlon.

Bonk A state of exhaustion that is reached in prolonged exercise when carbohydrate fuel stores are depleted.

Bottom bracket The short, horizontal cylinder that holds a bicycle crank axle.

Brake hoods The brake handle covers on standard road bicycle handlebars (known as drop handlebars). Brake hoods are usually referred to simply as "hoods."

Brick A workout in which a bike ride is followed immediately by a run.

Build phase The second of three phases in the training cycle, during which a triathlete maintains a consistent training volume while concentrating on high-intensity workouts.

Cadence The rate of pedaling on the bicycle, as expressed in revolutions per minute.

Capillaries Tiny blood vessels that allow for the exchange of gases and nutrients between blood and tissue cells.

Carbo loading A strategy that entails increasing dietary carbohydrate intake in the few days before a race to increase the amount of glycogen stored in the liver and muscles.

Cassette The set of toothed, circular cogs that sits on the rear hub of a bicycle. Also called a freewheel and a rear cluster. The smaller the cog a cyclist's chain is looped around at any given time, the higher a gear he or she is in.

Catch A phase of the arm stroke cycle in freestyle swimming, during which the swimmer creates a paddle with his or her hand and forearm in preparation for the pull phase.

Central fatigue A state that is characterized by inefficiency in the sending of movement signals from the brain and loss of the will to continue exercising and is precipitated by the depletion of blood glucose in the latter stages of workouts and competitions.

Chainring A circular, toothed cog attached to the right crankarm that turns with the pedals and drives the chain. Road and triathlon bikes have two chainrings, larger and smaller.

Chamois Bicycle shorts. Pronounced "shammy."

Crank The part of a bicycle that connects the pedal to the crank axle.

Crossover effect Fitness benefits that accrue in each of the three triathlon disciplines from training performed in the other two.

Cycle A repeating pattern of training. There are three levels of training cycle: weekly cycles, step cycles, and full training cycles.

Cyclometer A bicycle instrument that provides the rider with information such as current speed, trip distance, and trip time.

Dehydration A state in which the amount of water in the body has diminished below the level needed for optimal athletic performance.

Derailleur A mechanism that pushes the chain off of one sprocket and onto another in order to change the gear ratio. Road and triathlon bikes have two derailleurs, front and rear.

Detraining The gradual loss of fitness adaptations when training is reduced or ceases for a prolonged period of time.

DNF An acronym used in race results; it stands for "did not finish."

Drafting Gaining an energy advantage by following in the slipstream of another cyclist or swimmer. Bicycle drafting is illegal in most triathlons.

Drill A short-duration exercise involving a modified version of swimming, cycling, or running that is practiced for the sake of technique or power enhancement.

Duration The amount of time that an individual workout lasts.

Economy The relative energy efficiency of a swimmer, cyclist, or runner in motion.

Efficiency Another word for **economy.**

Electrolytes Mineral nutrients (sodium, chloride, magnesium, and potassium) that aid muscle contraction and nerve impulse transmission by conducting bioelectrical signals.

Endurance The ability to work at a relatively high intensity level for a long period of time.

Enzyme A protein that promotes one or more types of chemical reaction in the body without itself being altered.

Ergogenic aid A nutritional supplement that somehow assists or enhances energy production. Sports drinks and energy bars and gels are considered ergogenic aids.

Fartlek A type of running workout in which an athletes plays with his or her pace by whim.

Focus period A period during which a triathlete emphasizes training in one of the three triathlon disciplines.

Force An application of energy to generate movement or overcome resistance in a particular direction.

Free radical An unstable molecule, usually oxygen, that tends to damage living tissues in the body.

Frequency The total or average number of workouts a triathlete performs in a specified amount of time.

Functional strength training A form of strength training that simulates components of athletic movement patterns against resistance in order to increase the power with which an athlete is subsequently able to perform these movement patterns.

Glucose A sugar derived from dietary carbohydrate that serves as a primary muscle energy fuel during exercise.

Glycemic index A measure of how different foods affect blood glucose levels.

Glycogen A long chain of glucose molecules that is stored in skeletal muscle and the liver and serves as a primary muscle fuel source during exercise.

Hemoglobin A protein in the blood that transports oxygen to muscle cells.

Homeostasis A state of balance, or equilibrium, in a given system of the body.

Hub A bicycle wheel axle.

Hyponatremia A dangerously low concentration of sodium in the blood that can result from the combination of heavy perspiration and failure to ingest sodium during prolonged exercise.

Intensity The rate at which an athlete burns energy for movement relative to his or her maximum capacity to burn energy for movement in a given mode of exercise.

Interval A segment within a type of workout in which high-intensity efforts of a given distance or duration are separated by recovery periods of a specified duration. In cycling and running, it is usually the high-intensity segments that are called intervals, whereas in swimming, it is usually the combination of a single high-intensity swim effort and the subsequent rest period that is called an interval.

Ironman A trademark owned by the World Triathlon Corporation and a popular long-distance triathlon format comprising a 2.4-mile swim, 112-mile bike, and 26.2-mile run.

Jammers A type of swim shorts for men that fits tightly and covers the legs down to the kneecaps.

Jump A brief sprint performed by a group of cyclists during a training ride.

Kinesthetic awareness Awareness of the sensation of the body's position and movement in space.

Lactate threshold An intensity level of exercise above which the metabolic waste product lactic acid accumulates in the blood faster than the circulatory system can remove it. Also known as the **anaerobic threshold.**

Lactic acid A compound that is produced in the body primarily as a byproduct of anaerobic metabolism.

Lateral Refers to the outer sides (left and right) of the body.

Main set The longest (or only) interval set in a swim workout.

Max HR Short for maximum heart rate—that is, the highest heart rate one can achieve in swimming, cycling, or running.

Max oxygen Refers to training performed at 100 percent of VO_2 max or thereabouts.

Medial Refers to the center of the body.

Mitochondria Structures within cells that serve as the site of aerobic metabolism.

Mode A form of exercise. Triathlon contains three modes: swimming, cycling, and running.

Myoglobin A type of protein that is responsible for transporting oxygen molecules within muscle cells.

Overdistance Describes swim, bike, and run workouts of the greatest duration in one's training.

Overload A physical training stimulus that creates a need and opportunity for recovery and adaptation.

Overpronate Excessive medial rotation of the foot during the footstrike portion of the running stride.

Overtraining A ratio of training to rest that is insufficient to allow complete recovery from and adaptation to training stimuli.

Overuse injury Dysfunction in a bone, muscle, or other soft tissue generally resulting from heavy repetition of flawed movement patterns.

Pace One's rate of swimming, cycling, or running.

Paceline A single-file line of cyclists in training.

Passive recovery Recovery in the form of inactivity.

Peak A brief window of maximum athletic performance potential that occurs at the end of a complete training cycle and taper.

Peak phase The last of three phases in the triathlon training cycle, during which a triathlete focuses on performing highly race-specific workouts and getting adequate rest.

Periodization A training method that involves arranging various types of training in a sequence that will produce the highest possible level of fitness by the end of the cycle.

Phase A period of training that is characterized by a focus on certain specific types of training. There are three basic phases in triathlon training: base, build, and peak.

Posterior Refers to the rear side of the body.

Postural muscle A muscle that serves to hold a part of the body in a static position.

Power A combination of strength and speed.

PR Short for "personal record"—one's personal best time for a standard swimming, cycling, running, or triathlon race distance.

Prime mover A muscle that bears the heaviest workload in some movement pattern.

Quality Refers to a type of workout that emphasizes working at or above the anaerobic threshold.

Racing flats A very light type of running shoe used in racing and sometimes in quality workouts.

Recovery A process wherein one or more systems of the body returns to homeostasis following exertion.

Repetition A hard-effort segment within an interval or strength workout.

Rest A period of inactivity between segments of a workout or between workouts.

Saddle sore Sores on the groin or buttocks that are generally caused by pressure and friction during cycling, and sometimes subsequent infection.

Speed The ability to swim, cycle, or run quickly. Also, an intensity level of swimming, cycling, and running that is predominantly anaerobic and serves to improve economy, anaerobic metabolism, and lactic acid tolerance.

Speed work An interval-type running workout that emphasizes speed intensity and which usually takes place on a running track.

Spin To ride the bike at a moderate intensity level and a high pedaling cadence (85–95 RPM).

Split Short for split time—one's time for a segment of a workout or race. For example, in any triathlon, a participant records swim, bike, and run splits.

Sprint A brief spurt of maximum-intensity swimming, cycling, or running.

Stabilizer A muscle that acts to stabilize a moving joint or a non-moving part of the body during the performance of an athletic movement pattern.

Step cycle A two- to four-week period of training in which training volume is relatively high for the first week to three weeks and then drops during the final week for recovery.

Stride A running drill involving roughly 100 meters of running at one-mile race pace followed by a jogging recovery.

Supercompensation A synonym for **adaptation**.

Synergist A muscle that plays a secondary role in generating a certain movement.

T1 Short for "first transition." It refers to the swim-to-bike transition in a triathlon.

T2 Short for "second transition." It refers to the bike-to-run transition in a triathlon.

Taper A short period of light training that immediately precedes a peak race and is undertaken to allow the body to fully recover from and adapt to the preceding hard training.

Training log A dated journal in which a triathlete records training performed, race results, and other information pertinent to training.

Training schedule A calendar in which a triathlete plots information about anticipated workouts and races, usually leading up to a peak triathlon.

Transition Either of two parts of a triathlon where competitors change disciplines, first from swimming to cycling (T1), and then from cycling to running (T2).

Tri-bike Short for triathlon bike, a type of bike that is designed especially for the time-trial type of bike racing that occurs in triathlons.

Triglyceride The primary form of fat in the diet and the form in which fat is stored in the body. An important source of fuel during endurance exercise.

Tri-suit Short for triathlon suit, a performance garment that is designed to be worn through the swim, bike, and run portions of a triathlon.

Ventilatory threshold A level of exercise intensity where an athlete's body is consuming oxygen at its maximum rate.

VO$_2$ max The maximum rate at which a given athlete can consume oxygen.

Volume The total or average amount of training a triathlete performs within a specified period of time.

Wave A subgroup of triathletes within a larger field of race participants that is scheduled to start the race together at a certain time. Triathlons often start in waves to avoid overcrowding during the early portion of the swim.

Weekly cycle A recurring seven-day pattern of training.

Workload The total amount of energy a triathlete expends in training within a specified period of time. Workload is a function of training volume and intensity.

Appendix: Triathlon Resources

Governing Bodies

USA Triathlon
616 Monument St.
Colorado Springs, CO 80905
(719) 597-9090
www.usatriathlon.org
info@usatriathlon.org

USA Triathlon is the national governing body for the sport of triathlon
in the United States. Membership in USAT is required for participation
in all USAT-sanctioned events (the majority of triathlons in the U.S.).
A one-year membership costs $25.

USA Cycling
One Olympic Plaza
Colorado Springs, CO 80909
(719) 578-4581
www.usacycling.org
membership@usacycling.org

USA Cycling is the national governing body for the sport of cycling in the United States. Membership in USAC's road cycling branch, the United States Cycling Federation, is required for participation in all USCF-sanctioned road cycling events. A one-year membership costs $25.

USA Swimming
One Olympic Plaza
Colorado Springs, CO 80909
(719) 578-4578
memberservices2@usa-swimming.org
www.usa-swimming.org

USA Swimming is the national governing body for the sport of swimming in the United States. Membership in USAS is required for participation in all USAS-sanctioned events. Join through one of USAS's 59 local swim clubs. Fees vary from club to club.

USA Track & Field
One RCA Dome, Suite 140
Indianapolis, IN 46225
(317) 261-0500

USA Track & Field is the national governing body for the sports of track and field, long-distance running, and race walking in the United States. Membership benefits include accident insurance and discounts on running-related purchases from a variety of sources.

Other Organizations

League of American Bicyclists
1612 K Street Northwest, Suite 800
Washington, DC 20006-2802
(202) 822-1334
bikeleague@bikeleague.org
www.bikeleague.org

The League of American Bicyclists is the largest bicycling advocacy group in the United States. The organization works to promote bicycling-friendly communities throughout the country and to support bike safety programs.

Road Runners Club of America
510 North Washington St.
Alexandria, VA 22314
(703) 836-0558
office@rrca.org
www.rrca.org

The Road Runners Club of America is a national association of local running clubs. Member benefits include accident insurance and a bi-monthly magazine.

Triathlantic
www.triathlantic.com

Triathlantic is a Maryland-based triathlon association with members in 25 states in the eastern half of the U.S. It organizes races, offers coaching, and raises money for charities.

Event Calendar

Triathlete Magazine
2037 San Elijo
Cardiff, CA 92007
(760) 634-4100
www.triathletemag.com

Triathlete is the world's largest triathlon magazine. Each of the magazine's monthly issues contains an event calendar containing dozens of upcoming event listings. To subscribe to *Triathlete,* visit www.triathletemag.com and click on the "Subscribe Now!" link, or call (800) 441-1666.

You can also access a comprehensive online triathlon event calendar by logging on to triathletemag.com and then clicking on the "Calendar" link.

Event Registration Service

Active.com
www.active.com

Active.com is the world's largest participatory sports Web site. You can register for hundreds of triathlon, running, cycling, and other events in the United States and elsewhere, instantly and securely, using this convenient online service.

Triathlon Clubs

Triathlon clubs operate in almost every state, and many metropolitan areas have two or more to choose among. For a comprehensive listing of triathlon clubs nationwide, visit www.usatriathlon.org, click on "Clubs/Regions," and then click on "Find a Club."

Online Coaching Services

Mark Allen Online
www.markallenonline.com

Mark Allen Online is an automated online coaching engine designed by six-time Hawaii Ironman World Champion Mark Allen.

Multisports.com
www.multisports.com

Multisports.com offers a variety of distance coaching packages for triathletes of various types and budgets. Coaches include eight-time Hawaii Ironman World Champion Paula Newby-Fraser and *Triathlete* columnists Roch Frey and Paul Huddle.

Triathlon Academy
www.triathlonacademy. com

The Triathlon Academy offers a variety of distance coaching packages for triathletes of various abilities and budgets. The principal coach is former professional triathlete Troy Jacobson.

Triathlon Gold
www.trainright.com

Triathlon Gold offers a variety of distance coaching packages for triathletes of various abilities and budgets. Principal coaches are Canadian National Triathlon Teams Coach Lance Watson and three-time U.S. National Triathlon Champion Mike Pigg. The author of this book also coaches with Triathlon Gold.

Ultrafit
www.ultrafit.com

Ultrafit offers one-on-one distance coaching with a choice of coaches, who include Joe Friel, author of *The Triathlete's Training Bible,* and Gale Bernhard, author of *Training Plans for Multisport Athletes.*

Ironman Information

World Triathlon Corporation
www.ironmanlive.com

The World Triathlon Corporation is the parent company of Ironman, the premier name in long-distance triathlons. More than two-dozen official Ironman triathlons (2.4-mile swim, 112-mile bike, 26.2-mile runs) and other Ironman-affiliated triathlons take place around the world each year. All are qualifiers for the Hawaii Ironman World Championship, considered the Holy Grail of triathlon events, which occurs in Kailua Kona, Hawaii, in October. It is also possible to qualify for the Hawaii Ironman through a lottery. Visit www.ironmanlive.com or call for more information.

Triathlon Web Sites

Ironmanlive.com
www.ironmanlive.com

This is the official site of Ironman and provides a wide range of information and services, including training tips and links to the official Web sites of every Ironman qualifier. Also offered is live multimedia coverage of several Ironman events each year.

Slowtwitch.com
www.slowtwitch.com

This all-in-one triathlon Web site offers everything from race coverage to training advice and is especially noted for its product reviews and commentary.

Transition Times
www.transitiontimes.com

Transition Times is a news-oriented triathlon Web site that features timely worldwide race coverage.

Triathlete.com
www.triathlete.com

Not to be confused with the official Web site of *Triathlete Magazine,* triathlete.com is a good place to interact with and learn from others in the sport.

Triathlon Central
www.triathloncentral.com

This unique Web site maintains its own rankings of professional triathletes worldwide.

Trinewbies.com
www.trinewbies.com

Although ostensibly a resource for beginners, Trinewbies.com provides a wealth of training information that all triathletes can learn from and use.

Xtri.com
www.extremetri.com
This Australia-based Web site caters to long-distance specialists in the sport of triathlon.

Index